MW00618082

Notes

Rehabilitation Specialist's Pocket Guide

Dawn Gulick, PT, PhD, ATC, CSCS

Purchase additional copies of this book at your health science bookstore or directly from F. A. Davis by shopping online at www.fadavis.com or by calling 800-323-3555 (US) or 800-665-1148 (CAN)

A Davis's Notes Book

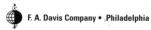

F. A. Davis Company • Philadelphia

F. A. Davis Company
1915 Arch Street
Philadelphia, PA 19103
www.fadavis.com

Printed in China by Imago

Last digit indicates print number: 10 9 8 7 6 5 4 3 2 1

Acquisition Editor: Margaret Biblis
Developmental Editor: Melissa Reed
Design Manager: Carolyn O'Brien
Reviewers: Lisa Dutton, PhD; David Krause, PT; James Laskin, PhD, PT; Corrie
Mancinelli, PhD, PT; Kristin Von Nieda, PT, DPT Med; Jaime C. Paz, PT, MS; Melissa
Peterson, PT, MHS, GCS; Nicholas Quarrier, BS, MHS; Laura Lee Swisher, PhD, PT;
Steven Tippett, PhD, PT, ATC, SCS; Frank B. Underwood, PhD, PT, ECS; Elizabeth L.
Weiss, PhD, PT, MS, CWS

Current Procedural Terminology (CPT) is copyright 2005 American Medical
Association. All Rights Reserved. No fee schedules, basic units, relative values, or
related listings are included in CPT. The AMA assumes no liability for the data
contained herein. Applicable FARS/DFARS restrictions apply to government use.

CPT® is a trademark of the American Medical Association.

Place $2\frac{7}{8} \times 2\frac{7}{8}$ **Sticky Notes** here

For a convenient and refillable note pad

✓ **HIPAA Supportive**
✓ **OSHA Compliant**

Waterproof and Reusable
Wipe-Free Pages

Write directly onto any page of *Screening Notes* with a ballpoint pen. Wipe old entries off with an alcohol pad and reuse.

Look for our other
Davis's Notes titles

Ortho Notes: Clinical Examination Pocket Guide
ISBN-10: 0-8036-1350-4 / ISBN-13: 978-0-8036-1350-8

Rehab Notes: Evaluation and Intervention Pocket Guide
ISBN-10: 0-8036-1398-9 /ISBN-13: 978-0-8036-1398-0

<u>Coming Fall 2006</u>

Derm Notes: Dermatology Clinical Pocket Guide
ISBN-10: 0-8036-1495-0 / ISBN-13: 978-0-8036-1495-6

ECG Notes: Interpretation and Management Guide
ISBN-10: 0-8036-1347-4 / ISBN-13: 978-0-8036-1347-8

LabNotes: Guide to Lab and Diagnostic Tests
ISBN-10: 0-8036-1265-6 / ISBN-13: 978-0-8036-1265-5

MedNotes: Nurse's Pharmacology Pocket Guide
ISBN-10: 0-8036-1109-9 / ISBN-13: 978-0-8036-1109-2

<u>New Edition Coming Fall 2006</u>

*For a complete list of Davis's Notes
and our other titles for health professionals, visit us online.*

For a complete list of Davis's Notes and other
titles for health care providers, visit
<u>www.fadavis.com</u>.

1

Organizational Sequence of This Manual

Tabs Across the Life Span

- Alerts & Alarms
- Pediatrics
- Adolescence
- Adult
- Pregnancy
- Geriatric

Within Each Tab

- Musculoskeletal
- Neuromuscular
- Cardiovascular/Pulmonary
- Integumentary
- Gastrointestinal
- Hepatic
- Endocrine
- Urogenital
- Additional information

What is a RED Flag?

Various pathologies are specific to gender, race, genetics, &/or occupation. Age may also place a person at a higher risk for the development of certain pathologies. Thus, this manual is arranged to cover the life span with this concept in mind. The clinician is encouraged to obtain a thorough history, complete a review of systems, clear adjacent structures, & then attempt to provoke the symptoms reported by the client. Failure to influence the symptoms of the client via palpation, motion, or the implementation of special tests should be a red flag for a pathological lesion that may lie outside the scope of the clinician's practice & require referral.

The term **red flag** is a common term used by a variety of health-care providers. However, there is not a universal definition of the term as common. For the purposes of this manual, a **red flag** will be defined as a sign or symptom that is a strong predictor of pathology or dysfunction of a particular organ system. Given a cluster of **red flags** that indicates a specific pathology, some **red flags** may be expected. For example, the complaint of chest pain for a known cardiac patient may be a common occurrence & may be less likely to trigger activation of emergency medical screening, identify **red flags**, sudden onset of chest pain & no cardiac history. Thus, it is up to the health-care provider to determine which **red flags** are appropriate to monitor and which should be acted upon immediately.

The purpose of this pocket guide is to help the health-care provider complete a thorough medical screening, identify **red flags**, & determine if the patient's needs are within the practitioner's scope of practice or if a referral would be appropriate. It is **not** designed to provide a differential diagnosis. It is the practitioner's responsibility to know the scope of his/her practice act.

Elements of Patient Management

This pocket guide will emphasize the first 3 elements of patient management:

- **Examination**—The process of obtaining a history, performing a review of systems, & administering tests/measures. This examination process may identify concerns that require consultation with or referral to another provider.
- **Evaluation**—The dynamic process of making clinical judgments based on the data from the examination.
- **Diagnosis**—The process of organizing the data into defined* clusters, syndromes, or categories.
- **Prognosis**—Determination of the level of optimal improvement that may be attained.
- **Intervention**—The purposeful and skillful interaction of the medical provider with the client to produce a change in the condition.
- **Outcome**—The result of patient management.

Source: Guide to Physical Therapist Practice.

Rationale for Screening

Leading Causes of Death for 2003

Adult	Children 1–14 yrs
■ Heart disease	■ Injury
■ Malignant neoplasms	■ Congenital
■ Cerebrovascular disease	malformations
■ Chronic lower respiratory	■ Malignant neoplasms
diseases	■ Homicide
■ Accidents	■ Heart disease
■ Diabetes mellitus	■ Suicide
■ Influenza & pneumonia	■ Pneumonia &
■ Alzheimer's disease	influenza
■ Nephritis & nephrosis	■ Septicemia
■ Septicemia	■ Benign neoplasms
■ Suicide	
■ Chronic liver disease & cirrhosis	
■ HTN & hypertensive renal disease	
■ Parkinson's disease	
■ Pneumonitis	

Source: National Vital Statistics Report, February 28, 2005.

Medical Screening

Have you ever experienced or been told you have any of the following conditions?

Cancer	Chronic bronchitis
Diabetes	Pneumonia
High blood pressure	Emphysema
Fainting or dizziness	Migraine headaches
Chest pain	Anemia
Shortness of breath	Stomach ulcers
Blood clot	AIDS/HIV
Stroke	Hemophilia
Kidney disease	Guillain-Barré syndrome
Urinary tract infection	Gout
Allergies (latex, food, drug)	Thyroid problems
Asthma	Multiple sclerosis
Osteoporosis	Tuberculosis
Rheumatic/scarlet fever	Fibromyalgia
Hepatitis/jaundice	Pregnancy
Polio	Hernia
Head injury/concussion	Depression
Epilepsy or seizures	Frequent falls
Parkinson's disease	Bowel/bladder problems
Arthritis	

Have you ever had any of the following procedures?

X-ray	Blood test(s)
CT scan	Biopsy
MRI	EMG or NCV
Bone scan	ECG or stress test
Urine analysis	Surgery

Screening for domestic violence:

Do you feel unsafe at home?
Has anyone in your home injured or tried to injure you?

Generalized Systemic Red Flags

- Insidious onset with no known mechanism of injury
- Symptoms out of proportion to injury
- No change in symptoms despite position, rest, or treatment
- Symptoms persist beyond expected healing time
- Recent or current fever, chills, night sweats, infection
- Unexplained weight loss, pallor, nausea, dizziness, vomiting, b&b changes (constitutional symptoms)
- Headache or visual changes
- Change in vital signs
- Bilateral symptoms
- Pigmentation changes, edema, rash, nail changes, weakness, numbness, tingling, burning
- Hx of cancer
- No pattern to the symptoms; unable to reproduce symptoms during the examination
- > 40 years old, gender, ethnicity, race
- Night pain
- Progressive neurology symptoms
- Cyclic presentation
- Joint pain with skin lesions
- (−) Waddell signs
- Psoas test for pelvic pathology = supine, SLR to 30° & resist hip flexion; (+) test for pelvic inflammation or infection is lower quadrant abdominal pain; hip or back pain is a (−) test
- Blumberg sign = rebound tenderness for visceral pathology
- (+) Kehr's sign (spleen) = violent Ⓛ shoulder pain
- Pain @ McBurney's point = 1/3 the distance from Ⓡ ASIS to umbilicus; tenderness = appendicitis

Signs/Symptoms of Emergency Situations

- SBP ≥ 180 mm Hg or ≤ 90 mm Hg
- DBP ≥ 110 mm Hg
- Resting HR > 100 bpm
- Resting RR > 30 bpm
- Sudden change in mentation
- Facial pain with intractable headache
- Sudden onset of angina or arrhythmia
- Abdominal rebound tenderness
- Black tarry or bloody stools

Normal Vital Signs & Pathologies That Influence Them

	Normal Values Across the Lifespan				Circumstances that may ↑ vital signs	Circumstances that may ↓ vital signs
	Infant	Child	Adolescent	Adult & Elderly		
T	98.2°	98.6°	98.6°	98.6°	Infection, exercise, ↑ blood sugar	↓ H&H, narcotics, ↓ blood sugar, aging
HR	80–180	75–140	50–100	60–100	Infection, ↓ H&H, CHF, ↑ blood sugar, COPD, fever, ↓ fluid volume, anxiety, anemia, pain, ↓ K⁺, exercise	Narcotics, acute MI, ↓ K⁺, beta blockers
RR	30–50	20–40	15–22	10–20	Infection, ↓ H&H, pain, ↑ blood sugar, anxiety, acute MI, asthma, exercise	Narcotics
SBP	73	90	115	< 130	CAD, anxiety, pain, exercise (SBP only)	↓ H&H, narcotics, acute MI, ↓ K⁺, cardiac meds, anemia
DBP	55	57	70	< 85	Renal disease, steroids, ↑ caffeine	

Cranial Nerves

Nerve	Function	Test
I. Olfactory	Smell	Identify odors with eyes closed
II. Optic	Vision	Test peripheral vision with 1 eye covered
III. Oculomotor	Eye mov't & pupillary reaction	Peripheral vision, eye chart, reaction to light
IV. Trochlear	Eye mov't	Test ability to depress & adduct eye
V. Trigeminal	Face sensation & mastication	Face sensation & clench teeth
VI. Abducens	Eye mov't	Test ability to abduct eye past midline
VII. Facial	Facial muscles & taste	Close eyes & smile; detect various tastes–sweet, sour, salty, bitter
VIII. Vestibulo-cochlear (acoustic)	Hearing & balance	Hearing; feet together, eyes open/closed x 5 sec; test for past-pointing
IX. Glosso-pha-ryngeal	Swallow, voice, gag reflex	Swallow & say "ahh" Use tongue depres-sor to elicit gag reflex
X. Vagus	Swallow, voice, gag reflex	
XI. Spinal Accessory	SCM & trapezius	Rotate/SB neck; shrug shoulders
XII. Hypoglossal	Tongue mov't	Protrude tongue (watch for lateral deviation)

Dermatomes

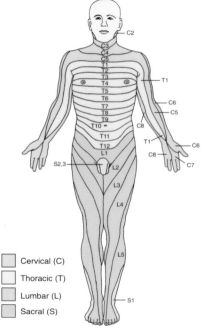

- Cervical (C)
- Thoracic (T)
- Lumbar (L)
- Sacral (S)

Source: Taber's Cyclopedic Medical Dictionary (2005).

Visceral Innervations & Referral Patterns

Segmental Innervation	Viscera	Referral Pattern(s)
C3–5	Diaphragm	C-spine & anterior shoulders
T1–5	Heart	Anterior neck, chest, Ⓛ UE
T3/4–6/7	Esophagus	Substernal & upper thorax
T5–6	Lungs	T-spine
T6–8	Spleen	Ⓛ shoulder & upper 1/3 of arm
T6–10	Stomach	Upper abdomen & T-spine
	Bile duct	Upper abdomen, mid T-spine
T7–10	Gallbladder	Ⓡ UQ, Ⓡ T-spine
	Liver	Ⓡ T-spine & Ⓡ shoulder
T5/6–10/11	Pancreas	Upper abdomen, low T-spine & upper L-spine
T7–10	Small intestine	Mid T-spine & umbilicus
T10–11	Testes/ovaries	Lower abdomen & sacrum
T10–12	Appendix	Ⓡ LQ, umbilicus
T10–L1	Kidney	High posterior costovertebral angle, radiates around flank
T10–L1	Uterus	L/S & T/L junction
S2–4	Prostate	Sacrum, testes, T/L junction
T11–L1	Bladder	Sacral apex, suprapubic & upper thighs
T11–L1	Large intestine	Lower abdomen, L-spine
T11–L2 S2–4	Ureter	Costovertebral angle, groin, suprapubic & medial thigh

Visceral Referral Patterns

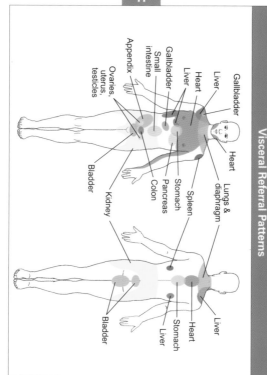

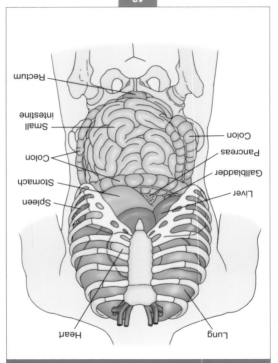

Visceral Diagrams

Rectum

Small intestine

Colon

Colon

Pancreas

Stomach

Gallbladder

Spleen

Liver

Heart

Lung

Visceral Palpation

Visceral pain is most often the result of:

- Hollow organ distention
- Ischemia
- Inflammation
- Muscle guarding
- Traction

Purpose:

Identify masses, tenderness, or irregularities

Technique

When deep palpation is impeded by muscle or adipose, use 2 hands. Place 1 hand on top of the other & apply pressure with the top hand while palpating with the bottom hand

Blumberg's Sign (Rebound tenderness for visceral pathology)

- In supine, select a site away from the painful area & place your hand perpendicular on the abdomen
- Push down slow & deep, hold for a moment then lift up quickly
- Red flag: (+) = pain on release; (–) = no pain

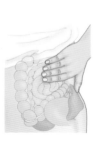

(Continued text on following page)

Visceral Palpation (Continued)

Murphy's Sign for the Gallbladder

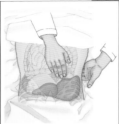

- Place fingers to ®) of rectus abdominis just below rib cage
- Ask patient to take a deep breath
- Red flag: Sudden pain & abdominal muscle tensing that ceases inspiration is suggestive of gallbladder pathology; pain also ↑ with FB

Spleen

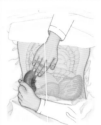

- With patient in supine, stand on the ®) & reach across with your Ⓛ hand to patient's ribs at the mid-axillary line
- Place ®) hand at the Ⓛ costal margin (fingers pointing to Ⓛ shoulder)
- Press in & up
- Ask patient to take an "abdominal" breath & the edge of the spleen will move toward your fingers
- Red flag: reproduction of symptom(s); if spleen is palpable, it is probably enlarged

(Continued text on following page)

Kehr's Sign for the Spleen

- With patient in supine, raise the foot of the bed (Trendelenburg position)
- Red flag: the presence of blood or other irritant in the peritoneal cavity will result in severe Ⓛ shoulder pain a few minutes after the LEs are elevated

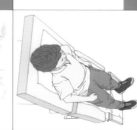

Liver Palpation

- With patient in supine, place Ⓛ hand under the patient parallel to 11th & 12th ribs & lift upward
- With your Ⓡ hand at the costal margin, lateral to the rectus (fingers pointing toward the clavicle), gently press up & in
- Ask patient to take an "abdominal" breath & you should feel the liver edge move toward your fingertips on the abdomen
- Follow the liver contour for irregularities & note tenderness
- Red flag: reproduction of symptom(s)

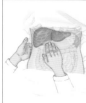

(Continued text on following page)

Visceral Palpation (Continued)

Right Kidney

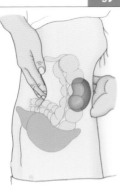

- With patient in supine, place Ⓛ hand under the patient between the ribs & iliac crest
- Place your Ⓡ hand on the abdomen just below the Ⓡ ribs with your fingers pointing Ⓛ
- Ask patient to take an "abdominal" breath & try to "capture" the Ⓡ kidney between your fingers
- Repeat with hands reversed for Ⓛ kidney
- Red flag: reproduction of symptom(s)

McBurney's Point for the Appendix

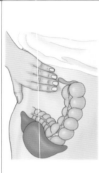

- In supine, identify the point that is half the distance between the Ⓡ ASIS & umbilicus
- Apply vertical pressure to this point
- Red flag: ↑ abdominal pain is a (+) test

(Continued text on following page)

Visceral Palpation (Continued)

Psoas Sign for Appendicitis

- In supine, place hand above pt's Ⓡ knee & resist hip flexion
- Alternate technique–in Ⓛ side-lying, hyperextend Ⓡ LE
- Red flag: ↑ abdominal pain is a (+) test

Obturator Sign for Appendicitis

- In supine, raise the pt's Ⓡ LE with the knee in flexion
- Perform IR of Ⓡ hip
- Red flag: ↑ abdominal pain is a (+) test

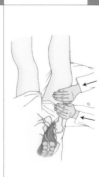

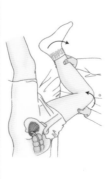

(Continued text on following page)

Visceral Palpation *(Continued)*

Aorta

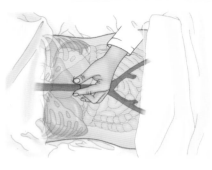

- Supine with hips/knees flexed
- At the upper abdomen, halfway between xiphoid & umbilicus, just Ⓛ of midline, press firm & deep to palpate the pulsation of the aorta
- Place your thumb on one side & your index/middle finger on the other side
- Palpate for a prominent lateral expansion of the aorta (aortic aneurysm)
- Alternate technique = use index/middle fingers of both hands
- Red flag: Aortic pulse width > 2 cm; back pain with palpation; bruit on auscultation

Source: Bates B (1995); Boissonnault WG (2005); Munro J & Campbell I (2000).

"CAUTIONS" = Red Flags of Cancer

- **C** = Change in bowel & bladder
- **A** = A sore that fails to heal in 6 weeks
- **U** = Unusual bleeding or discharge
- **T** = Thickening/lump (breast or elsewhere)
- **I** = Indigestion or difficulty swallowing
- **O** = Obvious change in wart or mole
  - **A** = Asymmetrical shape
  - **B** = Border irregularities
  - **C** = Color – pigmentation is not uniform
  - **D** = Diameter > 6 mm
  - **E** = Evolution (change in status)
- **N** = Nagging cough or hoarseness (rust-colored sputum)
- **S** = Supplemental signs/symptoms
  - + change in DTRs
  - + proximal muscle weakness
  - + night pain
  - + pathological fracture
  - > 45 years old

Signs & Symptoms of Specific Organ Pathology

Cardiac

- Chest pain*
- Irregular heartbeat (palpitations)
- Dyspnea, orthopnea
- Fainting, dizziness
- Rapid onset of fatigue

- Peripheral edema
- Cold hands/feet

- ↓ Peripheral pulse
- LE claudication
- Cyanotic nail beds

*Chest pain in individuals with known cardiac pathology may be stable angina & may not be a red flag for emergency care. Nitroglycerin, modification of activity, or monitoring of symptoms may be in order prior to seeking medical care.

Cardiac Auscultation

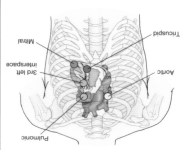

Aortic valve = 2nd intercostal space, (R) of sternum

Pulmonic valve = 2nd intercostal space, (L) of sternum

Tricuspid valve = 4th intercostal space, (L) of sternum

Mitral valve = 5th intercostal space @ midclavicular line

Labels on image: Tricuspid, Mitral, Aortic, Pulmonic, 3rd left interspace

Pulmonary

- Sharp, localized pain
- Fever, chills
- Symptoms aggravated by cold air or exertion
- ↓ Pain when recumbent; ↑ pain when lying on involved side
- Cough with/without blood
- Sputum
- SOB or DOE
- Crackles, wheezes, pleural friction rub on auscultation
- Clubbing of nails
- Wheezing
- Pain with deep inspiration
- ↑ O₂ saturation
- Weak/rapid pulse with ↑ BP = pneumothorax
- **Signs of PE:** pleural pain, SOB, ↑↑ RR & HR, coughing blood

Auscultation Pattern

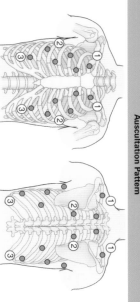

Adventitious Breath Sounds

- Bronchial breath sounds: louder than normal breath sounds
- Cavernous breath sounds: deep hollow sounds (like blowing over a bottle)
- Fine crackles: popping sound heard at the end of inspiration
- Course crackles: heard at the end of inspiration & disappear with cough
- Rhonchi: resembles snoring; obstructed or turbulent air flow
- Rales: clicking, bubbling, rattling sounds
- Wheezes: loud sounds that have a high-pitched musical quality; more easily detected with forced expiration
- Pleural rub: low-pitched coarse rubbing sound generally at the end of inspiration & beginning of expiration

Hepatic

- ® UQ pain
- Weight loss
- Ascites/LE edema
- Carpal tunnel symptoms
- Intermittent pruritus
- Weakness & fatigue
- Dark urine/clay-colored stools
- Asterixis (liver flap) = flapping tremor resulting from the inability to maintain wrist extension with forearm supported
- Jaundice/bruising; yellow sclera of the eye
- Pain referral to T-spine between scapula, ® shoulder, ® upper trap, ® subscapular region
- Palmar erythema (liver palms)
- White, not pink, fingernails

Endocrine

- Joint & muscle pain
- Paresthesia
- Dry, scaly skin
- Constipation
- Fatigue
- Dyspnea
- Brittle nails/hair
- Cold intolerance
- Weight change
- Periorbital edema
- Hoarseness
- Polydipsia/polyuria

Gastrointestinal

- Symptoms influenced by eating, swallowing
- Epigastric pain with radiation to the back
- Blood or dark, tarry stool
- Fecal incontinence/urgency, diarrhea/constipation
- Tenderness @ McBurney's point
- Pain that changes with eating
- Nausea, vomiting, bloating
- Food may help or aggravate px
- Weight loss, loss of appetite

Renal

- (+) Murphy's test = percussion over kidney
- Fever, chills
- Dull aching pain aggravated by prolonged sitting
- Blood in urine (hematuria)
- Cloudy or foul-smelling urine
- Painful or frequent urination
- Pain is constant (stones)
- Back pain at the level of the kidneys
- Costovertebral angle tenderness
- Skin hypersensitivity, pyuria
- HTN
- Bleeding tendencies; ecchymosis
- Headache
- Pruritus

Prostate

- Men > 50 yo with c/o LBP or suprapubic pain
- Difficulty starting or stopping urine flow
- Change in frequency; ↓ urine flow
- Nocturia, hematuria
- Incontinence/dribbling
- Sexual dysfunction
- PSA level > 4 ng/mL

Gynecological

- Cyclic pain
- Abnormal bleeding
- Nausea, vomiting
- Vaginal discharge
- Chronic constipation
- Low BP (blood loss)
- Missed or irregular periods
- Pain with cough/intercourse

Influence of Pathology on Lab Values

Test	↑	↓
RBC	■ Polycythemia ■ Renal disease ■ Pulmonary disease ■ CV disease	■ Anemia ■ Hodgkin's leukemia ■ Sickle cell disease
Hct (hematocrit) & Hgb (hemoglobin)	■ Dehydration ■ Shock ■ COPD ■ CHF ■ Polycythemia	■ Anemia ■ Leukemia ■ Hyperthyroidism ■ Cirrhosis ■ Massive trauma
WBC	■ Acute infection ■ Neoplasm ■ Leukemia	■ Bone marrow problem ■ Immunity problem ■ Iron deficiency, ETOH ■ Metastasis ■ Viral infection, AIDS ■ Chemotherapy
Erythrocyte Sedimentation Rate (ESR)	■ Kidney pathology ■ RA, lupus ■ Thyroid disease ■ Multiple myeloma ■ Inflammation ■ Pregnancy	■ CHF ■ Low plasma protein ■ Polycythemia ■ Sickle cell
Iron	■ Acute hepatitis ■ Nephrosis	■ Anemia ■ Lupus, RA ■ Hypothyroidism ■ 3rd trimester (pregnancy)
BUN	■ Kidney pathology ■ GI bleed ■ Heart failure ■ High-protein diet ■ Dehydration ■ Steroid use	■ Pregnancy ■ Malnutrition ■ Liver pathology ■ Acromegaly
Creatinine	■ Kidney pathology, hyperthyroidism	■ Loss of muscle mass ■ Aging

(Continued text on following page)

24

Influence of Pathology on Lab Values *(Cont'd)*

Test	↑	↓
Uric acid	■ Gout ■ Arthritis ■ Kidney stones/ disease	■ Chronic kidney disease ■ Low thyroid ■ Toxemia ■ ETOH
CPK	■ MI ■ ETOH ■ Skeletal mm disease	
LDH	■ MI, pulmonary infarct ■ Anemia, leukemia ■ Malignancy	■ Malnutrition ■ Hypoglycemia
GGT, AST/ SGOT ALT, SGPT	■ Liver pathology ■ Cardiac mm damage ■ ETOH ■ Muscle injury, MD ■ Neoplasm	■ Malnutrition ■ Vit B deficiency ■ Pregnancy ■ Hypothalamism ■ Hypothyroidism
Alkaline phos-phatase	■ Growing children ■ Pregnancy ■ Bone/liver pathology ■ Gallstones	■ Hypophosphatasia (genetic condition) ■ Hypoadrenia ■ Malnutrition
LDL	■ Atherosclerosis ■ CHD	■ Depression, anxiety ■ Violent behaviors, suicide ■ Hemorrhagic stroke
HDL	■ Vigorous exercise ■ Insulin ■ Estrogens	■ Starvation ■ Obesity, hypothyroidism ■ Smoking ■ DM, liver disease
T4	■ Hyperthyroidism ■ Pregnancy ■ Birth control pill	■ Hypothyroidism ■ Pituitary px

Electrolyte Imbalances

	Causes of ↓	Symptoms of ↓	Causes of ↑	Symptoms of ↑
Na⁺	■ Ketoacidosis ■ Diuretic use ■ Kidney disease ■ CHF ■ Vomiting/ diarrhea	■ H/A, confusion ■ Weakness, lethargy ■ Nausea, vomiting, diarrhea	■ Excess sweating ■ Hypothalamic ■ Diabetes ■ Hyperadrenalism	■ ↑Thirst; oliguria ■ Dry, flush skin ■ CNS-agitation ■ ↓DTRs & BP ■ Tachycardia ■ Weak, thready pulse
K⁺	■ Vomiting, diarrhea ■ Diuretic use ■ Corticosteroid use	■ Muscle cramps, weakness ■ Arrhythmias ■ Vomiting ■ SOB ■ ↑Thirst, polyuria	■ Diabetes ■ Adrenal insufficiency ■ Urinary obstruction	■ Muscle cramps, weakness ■ Nausea, diarrhea, GI distress ■ ECG changes
Ca⁺⁺	■ Vitamin D deficiency ■ Kidney disease ■ Hypoparathy- roidism	■ Paresthesia ■ Muscle cramps ■ ↑DTRs ■ Slow mental processing ■ (+) Chvostek test* ■ (+) Trousseau test**	■ Hyperparathy- roidism ■ Metastatic CA ■ Multiple myeloma	■ Muscle weakness; ataxia ■ Deep bone pain ■ HTN ■ Renal dysfunction ■ AV block on ECG ■ Nausea, vomiting, constipation

(Continued text on following page)

Electrolyte Imbalances (Continued)

	Causes of ↓	Symptoms of ↓	Causes of ↑	Symptoms of ↑
P	■ Hyperparathyroidism ■ Dietary	■ Intention tremor, ataxia ■ Paresthesia ■ ↓ DTRs ■ Muscle weakness ■ Joint stiffness ■ Bleeding disorder	■ Hypoparathyroidism ■ Hyperthyroidism ■ Kidney disease	■ ↑ BP ■ → Cardiac work ■ Risk of ↓ bone mineral density
Mg++	■ Dietary ■ DM ■ ETOH	■ Athetoid/choreiform mov'ts ■ (+) Babinski sign ■ Nystagmus ■ (+) Chvostek test* ■ (+) Trousseau test** ■ HTN, tachycardia (arrhythmia)	■ Dietary	■ Diarrhea ■ Nausea

*Chvostek test = Tap on side of face, below zygomatic arch, anterior to ear; (+) test = ipsilateral twitching of facial muscles.
**Trousseau test = Inflate sphygmomanometer above SBP for several minutes; (+) test = wrist, MCP, & thumb flexion with finger extension.

Source: Boissonnault WG (2005); Porth CM (1994).

Signs & Symptoms of Vitamin Deficiencies

Vitamin	Signs & Symptoms of Deficiencies
A	■ Eye px – ↑ night vision, dry eyes, inflammation ■ Rough/dry skin, folliculosis, gooseflesh ■ Vulnerability to respiratory/urinary infections ■ Failure of tooth enamel
B1 Thiamine	■ Tired, irritability, sleep px (beriberi) ■ Loss of appetite, vomiting ■ ↑ Muscle tone, hyperreflexia, nystagmus ■ Peripheral neuropathy & cardiac enlargement ■ Red burning tongue ■ LE edema ■ Wernicke's syndrome in ETOH
B2 Riboflavin	■ Cracked lips/corners of mouth (cheilosis) ■ Dermatitis, glossitis ■ Sore, magenta-colored tongue ■ Personality shifts
B3 Niacin	■ Pellagra = 4Ds: dermatitis, diarrhea, dementia, death ■ Bright red, painful, swollen tongue ■ Headaches, dizziness
B6 Pyridoxine	■ Anemia, weakness, diarrhea, wt loss ■ Irritability, depression, confusion, memory loss ■ Impaired antibody production, ↓ immunity ■ Kidney stones
B12 Cobalamin	■ Anemia ■ Poor resistance to infection ■ Nerve degeneration (needed for myelin) ■ Loss of LE position sense
C	■ Weakness, aches & pain (scurvy) ■ Swollen/bleeding gums, nosebleeds ■ Bruising easily (petechiae), poor healing ■ Anemia ■ ↑ Skeletal dev't in children

(Continued text on following page)

Signs & Symptoms of Vitamin Deficiencies *(Continued)*

Vitamin	Signs & Symptoms of Deficiencies
D	■ Osseous deformities (rickets), osteopenia ■ Bead-like swelling where ribs fuse with cartilage of the sternum
E	■ CNS changes ■ Liver degeneration ■ Anemia
K	■ Hemorrhage, ecchymosis ■ ↑ Blood clotting time

Signs & Symptoms of Diabetes

■ ↑ Urination
■ ↑ Thirst
■ ↑ Hunger

■ Fatigue, lethargy
■ Wt loss
■ Paresthesia (feet & hands)

Abnormal Blood Glucose

Hypoglycemia	Hyperglycemia
■ Blood glucose < 50–60 mg/dL ■ Skin is pale, cool, diaphoretic ■ Disoriented or agitated ■ Headache ■ Blurred vision ■ Slurred speech ■ Tachycardic with palpitations ■ Weak/shaky ■ Lip/tongue numbness ■ LOC	■ Blood glucose > 180 mg/dL ■ Skin is dry & flushed ■ Fruity breath odor ■ Blurred vision ■ Dizziness ■ Weakness ■ Nausea ■ Vomiting ■ Cramping ■ Increased urination ■ LOC/seizure

Headaches

Type of Pain	Possible Etiology
Acute	Trauma, infection, impending CVA
Chronic	Eye strain, ETOH, inadequate ventilation
Severe & intense	Meningitis, aneurysm, brain tumor
Throbbing/pulsating	Migraine, fever, hypertension, aortic insufficiency
Constant	Muscle contraction/guarding, with hx of HTN/anticoagulant = sentinel bleed
AM pain	Sinusitis (with d/c), ETOH, cervical DJD, hypertension, sleeping position
Afternoon pain	Eye strain, muscle tension
Night	Intracranial disease, nephritis
Forehead	Sinusitis, nephritis
Temporal	Eye or ear px, migraine, with visual changes = temporal arteritis
Occipital	Herniated disk, eye strain, hypertension
Parietal	Meningitis, constipation, tumor
Face	Sinusitis, trigeminal neuralgia, dental px, tumor
Stabbing pain	With ear fullness, tinnitus, vertigo = otitis media
Severe pain	With fever, + Kernig's sign = meningitis
Severe, sudden pain	Tumor, temporal arteritis, with ↑ BP = subarachnoid hemorrhage
Intermittent pain	With fluctuating consciousness = subdural hematoma
Postural	↑ Pain when upright & ↓ lying = dural tear

Visual Changes

Presentation	Possible Pathology
Loss of vision	Optic neuritis, detached retina, retinal hemorrhage, CNS px
Spots	Impending retinal detachment, fertility drugs
Floating spots	Diabetic retinopathy
Flashes	Migraine, retinal detachment
Visual field loss (shadows)	Retinal detachment, hemorrhage, macular degeneration
Photophobia	Iritis, meningitis
Distorted vision	Retinal detachment, macular degeneration/edema
Loss of vision in dim light	Myopia, vitamin A deficiency, retinal degeneration
Colored vision changes	Cataracts (colors seem faded), digitalis
Diplopia	Extraocular muscle paralysis, cataract
Loss of peripheral vision, haloes around lights	Glaucoma (ocular hypertension)
Hazy or protruding eye in a child	Congenital glaucoma
Cloudy or fuzzy vision	Cataracts

Amsler Grid

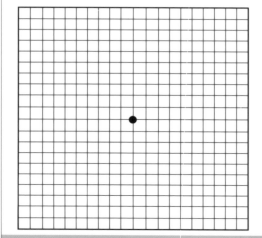

Instructions for Using the Amsler Grid

- Test your vision with adequate lighting
- Wear your glasses
- Hold the grid at normal reading distance (~14")
- Cover 1 eye at a time
- Stare at the center dot at all times
- Ask the following questions as you check each eye separately:
  - Are any lines crooked or bent?
  - Are any of the boxes different in size or shape?
  - Are any of the lines wavy, missing, blurry, or discolored?
- Report any irregularities to your eye doctor immediately

Nails	
Presentation	**Possible Pathology**
Beau's nails (transverse ridging)	Temporary arrest of nail growth due to a systemic insult, fever, infection, renal/hepatic px
Bitten nails	Anxiety
Clubbing	Respiratory/CV pathology, thyroid, ulcerative colitis, cirrhosis, CA
Curved	
Mees lines (white lines)	Arsenic poison, renal failure
Pitting (onycholysis)	Psoriasis
Red/brown distal nails	Renal failure
Red half-moons	CHF
Spoon nails (koilonychia)	Anemia, thyroid, syphilis, rheumatic fever
Splinter hemorrhages	Trauma, bacteria; endocarditis, MI
Terry's nails (white band)	Liver disease, sulfa drugs, antibiotics
Thick/crumbling	Fungal infection
Yellow	Bronchiectasis, thyroid disease, COPD, RA, malignancies, AIDS

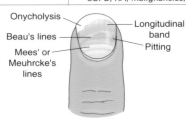

Source: From Barankin B & Freiman A (2006).

Skin

Presentation	Possible Pathology
Yellow jaundice–scleras	↓ Bilirubin 2° liver disease
Yellow carotenemia of palms/soles, face	Hypopituitarism, diabetes
Yellow uremia of skin	Chronic renal disease
Greenish-yellow	Obstructed bile ducts (↑ biliverdin)
Brown nipples, areolae, linea nigra, vulva	Pregnancy, Addison's disease, pituitary tumor
Bronze skin, genitalia	Hemochromatosis
Blue nails, lips	Hypoxia, cold exposure, heart disease, ↑ hemoglobin
Blue fingers	Raynaud's phenomenon
Reddish-blue face, mouth, hands/feet	Polycythemia
Red face, upper chest	Fever, ETOH, inflammation
Red	Carbon monoxide poisoning
Orange	Consumption of large quantities of carrots
Indigo discoloration	Gangrene, adrenal insufficiency
Violet-colored palms	Liver disease, pregnancy
Violet-colored LES	Cardiopulmonary compromise
Loss of color of skin, eyes, hair	Albinism, vitiligo, tinea versicolor

Locations of Dermatologic Conditions

FACE
Acne
Actinic keratosis
Basal cell carcinoma
Conatact dermatitis
Dermatomyositis
Herpes simplex
Impetigo
Keratoacanthoma
Lupus erythematosus
Melasma
Nevus
Perioral dermatitis
Rosacea
Sarcoidosis
Sebaceous hyperplasia
Seborrheic dermatitis
Seborrheic keratosis
Squamous cell carcinoma
Varicella-zoster infection
Vitiligo

LIMBS
Atopic eczema
Bullous pemphigoid
Cellulitis
Dermatofibroma
Erythema multiforme
Granuloma annulare
Henoch-Schonlein purpura
Keratosis pilaris
Lichen planus
Melanoma
Nevus
Psoriasis
Pyoderma gangrenosum
Seborrheic keratosis
Statis dermatitis
Ulcer
Vasculitis

GROIN
Candidal intertrigo
Erythrasma
Hailey-Hailey disease
Hydradenitis suppurativa
Psoriasis
Seborrheic dermatitis
Seborrheic keratosis
Skin tag
Tinea cruris

GENITALIA
Herpes simplex
Lichen planus
Lichen sclerosus
Molluscum contagiosum
Psoriasis
Scabies
Syphilis (chancre)
Wart
Zoon's balanitis

(Continued text on following page)

Locations of Dermatologic Conditions *(Continued)*

TRUNK

Acne
Basal cell carcinoma
Cherry angioma
Darier disease
Drug eruption
Epidermal cyst
Folliculitis
Grover disease
Keloid
Lipoma
Melanoma
Molluscum contagiosum
Morphea
Mycosis fungoides
Neurofibroma
Nevus
Pityriasis rosea
Psoriasis
Seborrheic keratosis
Skin tag
Striae
Syphilis
Tinea corporis
Tinea versicolor
Urticaria
Varicella-zoster infection

FEET

Contact dermatitis
Corn
Granuloma annulare
HFMD
Keratoderma
Lichen planus
Nevus
Onychomycosis
Plantar wart
Psoriasis
Tinea pedis

SCALP

Actinic keratosis
Alopecia areata
Androgenetic alopecia
Dermatitis
Epidermal or pilar cyst
Nevus
Pediculosis (lice)
Psoriasis
Seborrheic dermatitis
Squamous cell carcinoma
Tinea capitis

AXILLA

Acanthosis nigricans
Allergic contact dermatitis
Erythrasma
Hailey-Hailey disease
Hidradenitis suppurativa
Hyperhidrosis
Seborrheic dermatitis
Skin tag
Tinea corporis

HANDS

Actinic keratosis
Atopic eczema
Contact dermatitis
Erythema multiforme
Granuloma annulare
HFMD
Hyperhidrosis
Keratoacanthoma
Lichen planus
Psoriasis
Scabies
Syphilis
Warts

Source: From Barankin, B & Freiman A, (2006).

Sputum Analysis

Presentation	Possible Pathology
White	Bronchitis, CF
White & frothy	Pulmonary edema
Yellow–pale green	Infection
Rusty	Pneumonia
Foul-smelling	Anaerobic infection, lung abscess, CF, bronchiectasis
Hemoptysis	Pneumonia, acute bronchitis, lung CA, TB
Stringy mucus	After an asthma attack

Urinary Changes

Presentation	Possible Pathology
Red	Glomerulonephritis, TB, trauma, lupus, renal cystic disease
Orange/brown	Dehydration, ↑ bilirubin
Dark	Hepatic/bile obstruction, rhabdomyolysis
Milky/casts	Infection
Polyuria	Diabetes
↓ Flow	Obstruction, UTI, prostate hyperplasia
Fruity odor	Ketosis
Protein	Nephritis, DM, lupus, preeclampsia

Note: Some foods & meds can change urine color, e.g. beets, rhubarb, anticoagulants, sulfoamides.

Bowel Changes

Presentation	Possible Pathology
Melena (black, tarry)	Upper GI bleed (loss of > 150–200 mL of blood)
Black, non-sticky	Iron, bismuth salts (Pepto-Bismol), black licorice
Blood-red	Colon-rectal tumor, colon diverticulitis, hemorrhoids
Pale	↑ Fat absorption from small bowel, pancreatic disease
Silvery	Pancreatic cancer
Pencil-thin, ribbon stools	Distal colon/anal cancer

Signs & Symptoms of Depression

- Sadness; frequent/unexplained crying
- Feelings of guilt, helplessness, or hopelessness
- Suicidal ideations
- Problems sleeping
- Fatigue or decreased energy; apathy
- Loss of appetite; weight loss/gain
- Difficulty concentrating, remembering, & making decisions

Pain Assessment

Waddell Nonorganic Signs

Sign	Description
Tenderness—superficial or nonanatomic	Tenderness is not related to a particular structure. It may be superficial (tender to a light pinch over a wide area) or deep tenderness felt over a wide area (may extend over many segmental levels).
Simulation tests—axial loading in rotation	These tests give the client the impression that diagnostic tests are being performed. Slight pressure (axial loading) applied to the top of the head or passive rotation of the shoulders & pelvis in the same direction produces c/o LBP.
Distraction tests—SLR	A (+) clinical test (SLR) is confirmed by testing the structures in another position. By appearing to test the plantar reflex in sitting, the examiner may actually lift the leg higher than that of the supine SLR.
Regional disturbances—weakness or sensory	When the dysfunction spans a widespread region of the body (sensory or motor) that cannot be explained via anatomical relationships. This may be demonstrated by the client "giving way" or cogwheel resistance during strength testing of many major muscle groups or reporting diminish sensation in a nondermatomal pattern (stocking effect).
Overreaction	Disproportionate responses via verbalization, facial expressions, muscle tremors, sweating, collapsing, rubbing affected area, or emotional reactions.

Note: Any positive test in 3 or more categories results in an overall positive Waddell Score.

Source: Waddell G. (1980).

Ransford Pain Drawings

Indicate where your pain is located & what type of pain you feel at the present time. Use the symbols below to describe your pain. Do not indicate areas of pain that are not related to your present injury or condition.

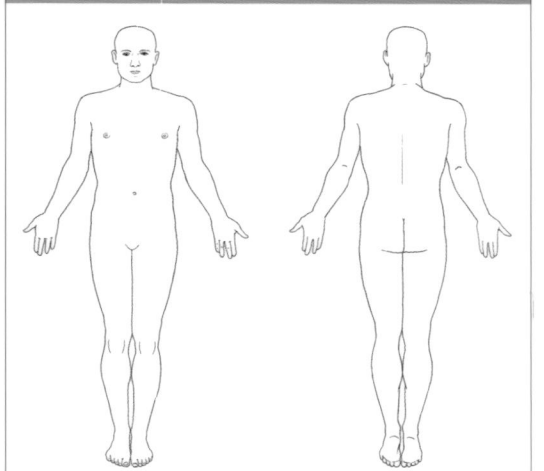

| /// | Stabbing | XXX | Burning |
| 000 | Pins & Needles | = = = | Numbness |

Source: From Gulick, D (2005).

Ransford Scoring System:

- Unreal drawings (score 2 points for any of the following)
  - Total leg pain
  - Front of leg pain
  - Anterior tibial pain
  - Back of leg & knee pain
  - Circumferential thigh pain
  - Lateral whole leg pain
  - Bilateral foot pain
  - Circumferential foot pain
  - Anterior knee & ankle pain
  - Scattered pain throughout whole leg
  - Entire abdomen pain
- Drawings with "expansion" or "magnification" of pain (1–2 points)
  - Back pain radiating into iliac crest, groin, & anterior perineum
  - Pain drawn outside of diagram
- Additional explanations, circles, lines, arrows (1 point each)
- Painful areas drawn in (score 1 for small areas & 2 for large areas)

Interpretation: A score of 3 or more points is thought to represent a pain perception that may be influenced by psychological factors.

Scoring:

Source: Ransford AO, Cairns D, & Mooney V (1976).

Short Form McGill Pain Questionnaire

Instructions: Read the following descriptions of pain and mark the number that indicates the level of pain you feel in each category according to the following scale:

1 = None   2 = Mild   3 = Moderate   4 = Severe

Throbbing	
Shooting	
Stabbing	
Sharp	
Cramping	
Gnawing	
Hot–Burning	
Aching	
Heavy	
Tender	
Splitting	
Tiring/Exhausting	
Sickening	
Fearful	
Punishing/Cruel	

Total Score: _____

The higher the score, the more intense the pain.

Source: Melzack R (1983); Melzack R (1987).

Present Pain Intensity Index

Instructions: Use the descriptors below to indicate your current level of pain.

0 = No Pain
1 = Mild
2 = Discomforting
3 = Distressing
4 = Horrible
5 = Excruciating

Substance Abuse

Risks of Pathology Associated with Tobacco

- CVD, PVD, COPD
- Tobacco amblyopia
- Carcinoma of mouth
- Lung cancer
- Peptic ulcer
- Small babies; obstetric or fertility problems
- ↑ Risk of bladder cancer
- ↑ Risk of kidney cancer
- ↑ Risk of breast cancer
- ↑ Risk of cervical cancer (♀)
- Addiction
- Poor recovery from LBP, Sx
- Impaired insulin absorption
- Premature aging
- **Children of smokers =** ↑ Respiratory px, ↑ ear infections & ↑ risk of fires

Source: American Cancer Society (1999); Munro J & Campbell I (2000).

Risks of Pathology Associated with Caffeine

- ↑ Blood sugar, ↑ blood fats, ↑ BP
- Stimulates CNS—tremors, irritability, nervousness
- Irregular heart beat
- ↑ Urinary Ca^{++} & Mg^{++} losses (↓ bone mineralization)
- ↑ Stomach acid secretion
- Disrupted sleep patterns—anxiety & depression
- ↑ Symptoms of PMS

Source: Andrews University Nutrition Department.

Caffeine Content (mg)

- Coffee = 110–150
- Decaf coffee = 2–5
- Tea = 9–50
- Cocoa = 6–35
- Regular & Diet—Mountain Dew, Mello Yellow, TAB, Coke, Pepsi, Mr. Pibb, Dr. Pepper = 36–54
- Red Bull = 80
- Anacin = 32
- Excedrin = 65
- Midol = 32
- Dexatrim = 200
- Darvon Compound = 32
- Vivarin = 200
- NoDoz = 100

Source: Gatorade Sports Science Institute (1990).

Substance Abuse Questionnaire	YES	NO
1. Have you ever decided to stop drinking for a week or so, but only lasted for a couple of days?		
2. Do you wish people would mind their own business about your drinking—stop telling you what to do?		
3. Have you ever switched from one kind of drink to another in the hope that this would keep you from getting drunk?		
4. Have you had to have an eye-opener upon awakening during the past year?		
5. Do you envy people who can drink without getting into trouble?		
6. Have you had problems connected with drinking during the past year?		
7. Has your drinking caused trouble at home?		
8. Do you ever try to get "extra" drinks at a party because you do not get enough?		
9. Do you tell yourself you can stop drinking any time you want to, even though you keep getting drunk when you don't mean to?		
10. Have you missed days of work or school because of drinking?		
11. Do you have "blackouts"?		
12. Have you ever felt that your life would be better if you did not drink?		

≥ 4 YES answers may indicate the need for substance abuse counseling

Source: Is AA for you? (1973).

Risks of Pathology Associated with Alcohol

- Alcoholic dementia
- Subdural hematoma from falls
- Convulsions from withdrawal
- Delirium tremens
- Cardiomyopathy

- Hypertension
- Hepatic cirrhosis
- Pancreatitis
- Dupuytren's contracture
- Myopathy
- Peripheral neuropathy

Source: Munro J & Campbell I (2000).

Risks of Pathology Associated with Obesity

- Arteriosclerosis, hypertension, CVA, & MI
- Sleep apnea
- Hypoventilation & exertional breathlessness
- Gallstones
- Diabetes

- Reflux
- OA
- Abdominal striae & varicose veins
- Impaired fertility
- Dependent edema

Body Mass Index (BMI)

$$\frac{\text{Weight in pounds} \times 700}{(\text{Height in inches})^2} = \text{BMI}$$

BMI	Classification
< 18	Underweight
18-25	Normal
26-29	Overweight
30-39	Obese
≥ 40	Morbid obesity

Note: BMI is a simple method to assess the possibility of health risks associated with obesity. BMI addresses weight relative to height & does NOT consider body composition. The gold standard for the assessment of obesity is % body fat determined via underwater weighing.

Growth Charts

■ Pediatric Head Circumference–Females

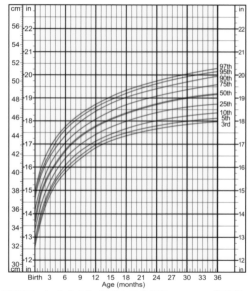

Age (months)

SOURCE: Developed by the National Center for Health Statistics in collaboration with the National Center for Chronic Disease Prevention and Health Promotion (2002).

Center for Disease Control

Source: http://www.kidsgrowth.com/stages/viewgrowthcharts. cfm?id = GH036

■ Pediatric Height Charts–Females: Birth to 36 months

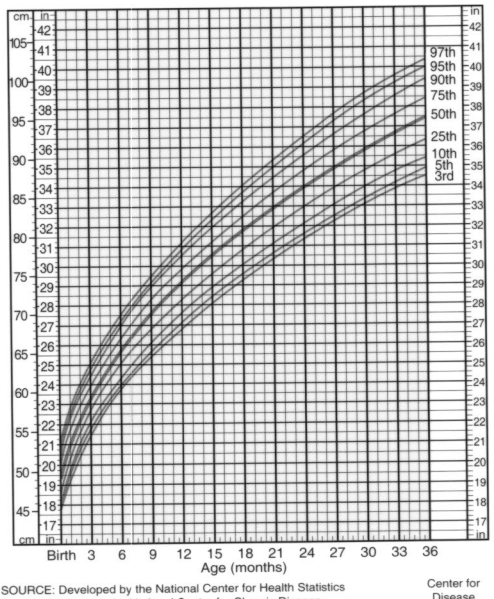

SOURCE: Developed by the National Center for Health Statistics in collaboration with the National Center for Chronic Disease Prevention and Health Promotion (2002).

Center for Disease Control

Source: http://www.kidsgrowth.com/stages/viewgrowthcharts.cfm?id=GH036

Growth Charts (Continued)

- Pediatric Weight Charts–Females: Birth to 36 months

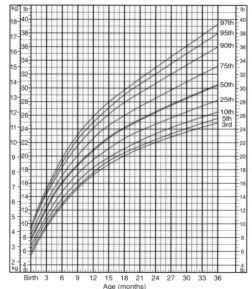

SOURCE: Developed by the National Center for Health Statistics in collaboration with the National Center for Chronic Disease Prevention and Health Promotion (2002).

Center for Disease Control

Source: http://www.kidsgrowth.com/stages/viewgrowthcharts. cfm?id=GH036

Growth Charts (Continued)

■ Pediatric Head Circumference–Males

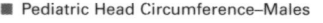

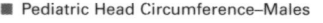

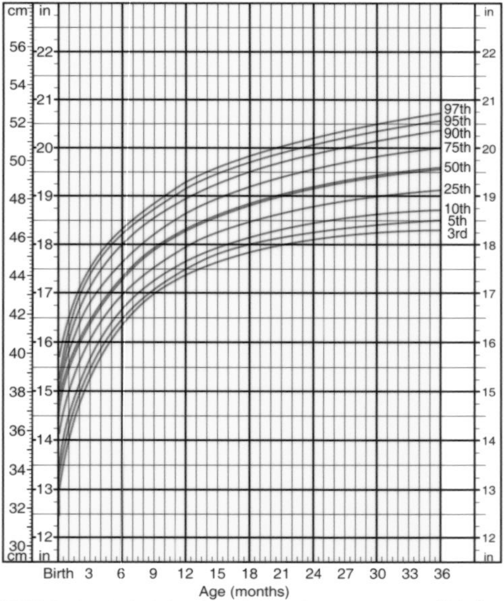

SOURCE: Developed by the National Center for Health Statistics in collaboration with the National Center for Chronic Disease Prevention and Health Promotion (2002).

Center for Disease Control

Source: http://www.kidsgrowth.com/stages/viewgrowthcharts. cfm?id=GH036

Growth Charts (Continued)

■ **Pediatric Height Charts–Males: Birth to 36 months**

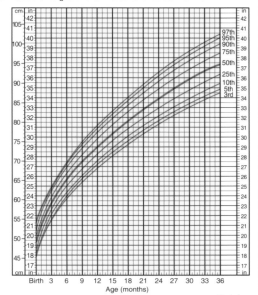

Age (months)

SOURCE: Developed by the National Center for Health Statistics
in collaboration with the National Center for Chronic Disease
Prevention and Health Promotion (2002).

Source: http://www.kidsgrowth.com/stages/viewgrowthcharts.
cfm?id = GH036

Center for
Disease
Control

■ Pediatric Weight Charts–Males: Birth to 36 months

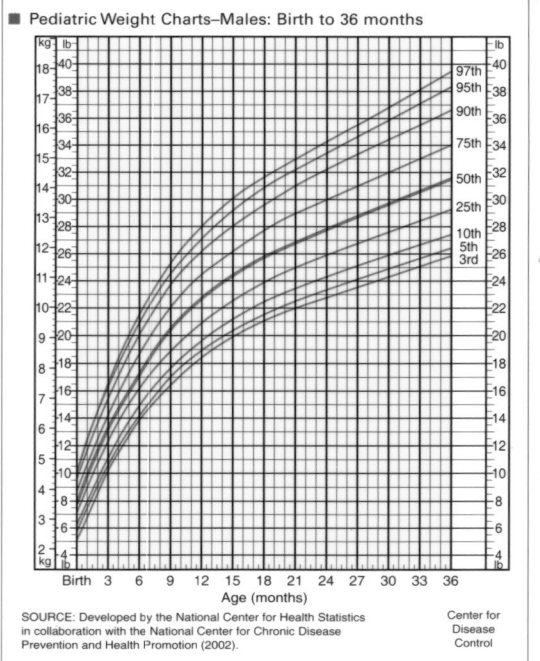

SOURCE: Developed by the National Center for Health Statistics
in collaboration with the National Center for Chronic Disease
Prevention and Health Promotion (2002).

Center for
Disease
Control

Source: http://www.kidsgrowth.com/stages/viewgrowthcharts.
cfm?id=GH036

Growth Charts *(Continued)*

■ Pediatric Height Charts–Females: 2–20 years

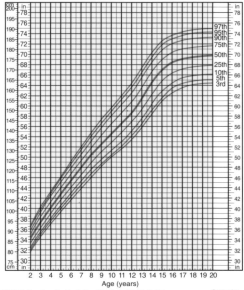

Age (years)

SOURCE: Developed by the National Center for Health Statistics in collaboration with the National Center for Chronic Disease Prevention and Health Promotion (2002).

Center for Disease Control

Source: http://www.kidsgrowth.com/stages/viewgrowthcharts. cfm?id=GH036

Growth Charts (Continued)

■ Pediatric Weight Charts–Females: 2–20 years

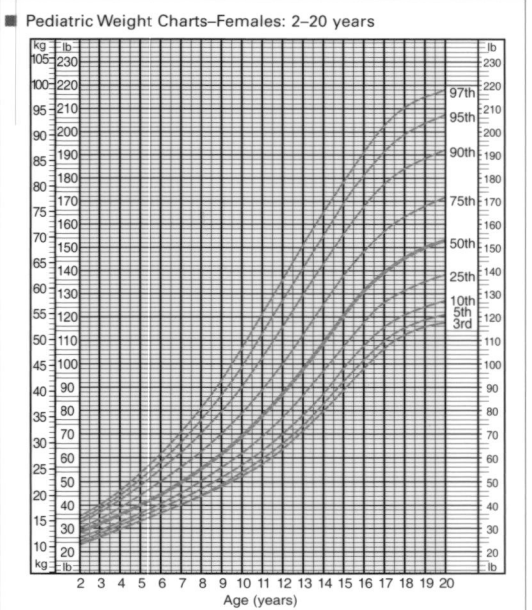

Age (years)

SOURCE: Developed by the National Center for Health Statistics in collaboration with the National Center for Chronic Disease Prevention and Health Promotion (2002).

Center for Disease Control

Source: http://www.kidsgrowth.com/stages/viewgrowthcharts. cfm?id=GH036

Growth Charts (Continued)

■ Pediatric Height Charts–Males: 2–20 years

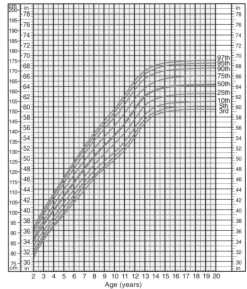

SOURCE: Developed by the National Center for Health Statistics in collaboration with the National Center for Chronic Disease Prevention and Health Promotion (2002).

Center for Disease Control

Source: http://www.kidsgrowth.com/stages/viewgrowthcharts.cfm?id = GH036

■ Pediatric Weight Charts–Males: 2–20 years

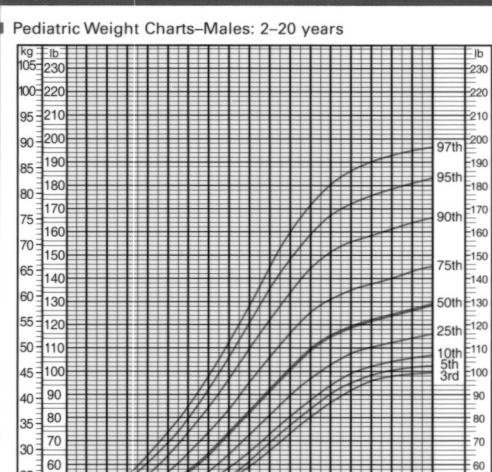

Age (years)

SOURCE: Developed by the National Center for Health Statistics in collaboration with the National Center for Chronic Disease Prevention and Health Promotion (2002).

Center for Disease Control

Source: http://www.kidsgrowth.com/stages/viewgrowthcharts. cfm?id=GH036

Pediatric Vital Signs

	HR	RR	SBP
Newborn (< 1 yr)	100–160	30–60	> 60
Toddler (1–3 yrs)	90–150	24–40	> 70
Preschooler (4–5 yrs)	80–140	22–34	> 75
Elementary (6–12 yrs)	70–120	18–30	> 80

		SBP (mm Hg) ♂			DBP (mm Hg) ♂		
		Percentile of Height			Percentile of Height		
Age	BP %-tile	5th	50th	95th	5th	50th	95th
1	50th	80	85	89	34	37	39
	95th	98	103	106	54	56	58
2	50th	84	88	92	39	42	44
	95th	101	106	110	59	61	62
3	50th	86	91	95	44	46	48
	95th	104	109	113	63	65	67
4	50th	88	93	97	47	50	52
	95th	106	111	115	66	69	71
5	50th	90	95	98	50	53	55
	95th	108	112	116	69	72	74
6	50th	91	96	100	53	55	57
	95th	109	114	117	72	74	76
7	50th	92	97	101	55	57	59
	95th	110	115	119	74	76	78
8	50th	94	99	102	56	59	61
	95th	111	116	120	75	78	80
9	50th	95	100	104	57	60	62
	95th	113	118	121	76	79	81
10	50th	97	102	106	58	61	63
	95th	115	119	123	77	80	82

Age	BP %-tile	SBP (mm Hg) ♂			DBP (mm Hg) ♀		
		Percentile of Height			Percentile of Height		
		5th	50th	95th	5th	50th	95th
1	95th	100	104	107	56	58	60
	50th	83	86	90	38	40	42
2	95th	102	105	109	61	63	65
	50th	85	88	91	43	45	47
3	95th	104	107	110	65	67	69
	50th	86	89	93	47	49	51
4	95th	105	108	112	68	70	72
	50th	88	91	94	50	52	54
5	95th	107	110	113	70	72	74
	50th	89	93	96	52	54	56
6	95th	108	111	115	72	74	76
	50th	91	94	98	54	56	58
7	95th	110	113	116	73	75	77
	50th	93	96	99	55	57	59
8	95th	112	115	118	75	76	78
	50th	95	98	101	57	58	60
9	95th	114	117	120	76	77	79
	50th	96	100	103	58	59	61
10	95th	116	119	122	77	78	80
	50th	98	102	105	59	60	62

Developmental Reflexes–Primitive/Spinal

Reflex	Stimuli	Expression	Integration*
Crossed extension	Noxious stimuli to ball of foot	28 wks gestation	1–2 months
Flexor withdrawal	Noxious stimuli to sole of foot	28 wks gestation	1–2 months
Rooting	Touch cheek	28 wks gestation	3 months
Suck-swallow	Object in mouth	28 wks gestation	2–5 months
Traction	Grasp forearm to pull up	28 wks gestation	2–5 months
Moro	Ext&ab of UE w/position change	28 wks gestation	5–6 months
Plantar grasp	Pressure to ball of foot	28 wks gestation	9 months
Galant	Infant turns when stroked	32 wks gestation	2 months
Positive supporting	Rigid WB with foot contact	32 wks gestation	1–2 months
Spont stepping	Stepping mov'ts in supine	37 wks gestation	2 months
Tonic lab	Prone = ↑ flex & supine = ↑ ext	Birth	6 months

*Integration is defined as the time in which the reflex is no longer dominant. Reflexive posturing may still present during the acquisition of new skills & in times of stress.

Developmental Reflexes—Tonic/Brain Stem

Reflex	Stimuli	Expression	Integration*
ATNR	Head rotation = fencing posture	Birth–2 months	4–6 months
Palmar grasp	Pressure to palm of hand	Birth–2 months	4–6 months
Lab head righting	Head orients when face is tipped	32 wks	5–6 months
Landau	Prone–arches back to raise head	3–4 months	12–24 months
STNR	Neck flexion/extension	4–6 months	10–12 months
Neck righting	Rotate head = body rotates	4–6 months	5 yrs
Body righting	Rotation of body	4–6 months	4–5 yrs
Instinctual grasp	Close hand to pressure	4–11 months	Life
Tilting–prone	Aligns body when tilted	6 months	Life
Protective ext–FW	UEs respond to COG outside BOS	6–7 months	Life
Protective ext–side	UEs respond to COG outside BOS	7 months	Life
Tilting–supine	Aligns body when tilted	7–8 months	Life
Tilting–sitting	Aligns body when tilted	7–8 months	Life
Protective ext–BW	UEs respond to COG outside BOS	9–10 months	Life
Tilting–quadruped	Aligns body when tilted	9–12 months	Life
Tilting– standing	Aligns body when tilted	12–21 months	Life
Protective staggering	LEs respond to COG outside BOS	15–18 months	Life

*Integration is defined as the time in which the reflex is no longer dominant. Reflexive posturing may still present during the acquisition of new skills & in times of stress.

Developmental Milestones

Age	Physical	Sensory/Cognitive
1 month	■ Reflex mov't ■ Brings hands to face ■ Lifts head briefly	■ Hearing is mature ■ Focuses @ 8–12"
2 months	■ Lifts head ■ Hands in fist	■ Smiles ■ Tracks with eyes ■ "Ah" & "Ooh" sounds
3 months	■ Turns prone to side ■ Sits with support ■ Brings hands together ■ Wiggles/kicks in supine ■ Reaches for objects ■ Grasps/shakes toys ■ Opens/shuts hand ■ Pushes down w/LE when feet are on ground	■ Cries to communicate hunger, fear, discomfort ■ Anticipates being lifted ■ Turns toward colors
4 months	■ Turns prone to supine ■ Supports upper body with arms in prone ■ Holds head erect	■ Makes consonant sounds ■ Laughs
5 months	■ Turns supine to prone ■ Plays with toes	
6 months	■ Reaches/grasps objects ■ Helps hold bottle ■ Moves toys between hands ■ Pulls up to sit ■ Sits with UE support ■ Rolls over ■ Bounces in standing	■ Opens mouth for spoon ■ Babbles ■ Laughs ■ Smiles in mirror ■ Knows familiar faces ■ Plays "peak-a-boo"
8 months	■ Pulls to stand ■ Sits without support ■ Explores with hands & mouth ■ Raking grasp	■ Fear of strangers ■ Responds to expressions ■ Tracks moving objects

(Continued text on following page)

Developmental Milestones (Continued)

Age	Physical	Sensory/Cognitive
9 months	■ Cruises along furniture ■ Well-developed crawl	■ Drinks from cup ■ Attempts to feed self ■ Looks for hidden objects
12 months	■ Walks alone or 1 hand held ■ Falls frequently when walking ■ Points with 1 finger ■ Pulls off socks ■ Crawl forward on belly ■ Creeps on hand/knees ■ Assumes quadruped	■ Drinks well from cup ■ Apprehensive with strangers ■ Cries when parent leaves ■ Says "dada" & "mama" ■ Responds to music with motion
18 months	■ Turns pages in a book ■ Carries a stuffed animal or doll ■ Stacks 2 blocks ■ Pulls off hat, socks, mittens ■ Scribbles with crayons ■ Runs clumsily ■ Jumps in place	■ Looks for hidden objects ■ Follows 1-step directions ■ 8-10 word vocabulary ■ Points/asks for things
24 months	■ Picks up toys without falling ■ Takes steps backward ■ Walks up steps with help ■ Kicks a ball ■ Pulls toy when walking ■ Scribbles ■ Climbs on furniture ■ Tosses/rolls a ball ■ Feeds self with spoon	■ 2- to 3-word sentences ■ Imitates parents ■ Treats doll stuffed animal as if live ■ Points to body parts when asked ■ Enjoys looking at a book repeatedly ■ Sometimes gets angry

(Continued text on following page)

Developmental Milestones *(Continued)*

Age	Physical	Sensory/Cognitive
3 years	■ Climbs ■ Walks up/down stairs with alternating feet ■ Runs ■ Pedals a tricycle ■ Bends down without falling ■ Turns 1 page @ a time ■ Holds pencil correctly ■ Opens/closes jars ■ Stacks 6 blocks ■ Rotates handles	■ Follows 2- to 3-step commands ■ Uses 4- to 5-word sentences ■ Expresses affection ■ Separates from parents ■ Sorts by color/shape ■ Pretends ■ Plays with mechanical toys ■ Takes turns
4 years	■ Hops on 1 foot ■ Throws ball overhand ■ Catches/bounces ball ■ Uses scissors ■ Draws circles/squares ■ Copies some letters ■ Dresses/undresses	■ Names colors ■ Starts counting ■ Begins problem-solving ■ Imagines monsters ■ Negotiates solutions to conflict
5 years	■ Stands on 1 foot x 10 seconds ■ Somersaults ■ Swings & climbs ■ May skip ■ Draws a person ■ Prints some numbers ■ Uses fork & spoon ■ Cares for toilet needs	■ Counts > 10 ■ Knows > 4 colors ■ Sentences > 5 words ■ Develops friendships ■ Agrees to rules ■ Sings & dances ■ Aware of gender ■ Expresses emotions

Maturation of Gait

9–15 Months

- "High guard"
- Hip flexion, abduction & ER
- Genu varum
- Flat feet
- No heel strike
- Wide BOS
- No trunk rotation
- Lateral wt shifts
- Limited single-leg stance

18–24 Months

- Begins to heel strike but still minimal push-off
- Increasing trunk rotation
- Increasing stride length
- Decreased genu varum
- Begins to include arm swing

3–4 Years

- Mild genu valgum
- Increasing pelvic rotation
- Notable wt shifting
- BOS = width of pelvis

6–7 Years

- Reciprocal arm swing
- Narrow BOS
- Heel strike & push-off
- Horizontal translation > vertical

Standing Balance Norms

Tandem

Eyes open = 29 ± 2 sec	Eyes closed = 23 ± 10 sec

Single-leg stance

Eyes open = 28 ± 4 sec	Eyes closed = 13 ± 10 sec

Source: Gagnon I, Swaine B, Friedman D & Forget R (2004); Atwater SW, Crowe TK, Deitz JC & Richardson PK (1990).

Pediatric Balance Scale

In every section, mark the 1 response that most closely describes the child's best performance in 3 attempts:

1. **Sitting to standing**—"Hold arms up & stand up"
   — Able to stand without using hands & stabilize independently
   — Able to stand independently using hands
   — Able to stand using hands after several tries
   — Needs minimal assist to stand or stabilize
   — Needs moderate or maximal assist to stand

2. **Standing to sitting**—"Sit down slowly without using your hands"
   — Sits safely with minimal use of hands
   — Controls descent by using hands
   — Uses back of legs against chair uncontrol descent
   — Sits independently, but has uncontrolled descent
   — Needs assistance to sit

3. **Transfers**—"Child transfers 1-way to a seat with armrest & 1-way to a seat without armrests"
   — Able to transfer safely with minor use of hands
   — Able to transfer safely; definite need of hands
   — Able to transfer with verbal cueing &/or supervision
   — Needs 1 person to assist
   — Needs 2 people to assist or supervise (close guard) to be safe

4. **Standing unsupported**—"Stand 30 seconds without holding on or moving his/her feet"
   — Able to stand safely 30 seconds
   — Able to stand 30 seconds w/supervision
   — Able to stand 15 seconds unsupported
   — Needs several tries to stand 10 seconds unsupported
   — Unable to stand 10 seconds unassisted

(Continued text on following page)

Pediatric Balance Scale (Continued)

5. Sitting with back unsupported & feet on floor—"Sit with arms folded on chest for 30 seconds"
— Able to sit safely & securely 30 seconds
— Able to sit safely & securely 30 seconds under supervision or may require use of arms to maintain sitting position
— Able to sit 15 seconds
— Able to sit 10 seconds
— Unable to sit 10 seconds without support

6. Standing unsupported with eyes closed—"Stand still, close eyes, & keep them closed"
— Able to stand 10 seconds safely
— Able to stand 10 seconds with supervision
— Able to stand 3 seconds
— Unable to keep eyes closed 3 seconds but stays steady
— Needs help to keep from falling

7. Standing unsupported with feet together—"Place feet together & stand still without holding on"
— Able to place feet together independently & stand 30 seconds safely
— Able to place feet together independently & stand for 30 seconds with supervision
— Able to place feet together independently but unable to hold for 30 seconds
— Needs help to attain position but able to stand 30 seconds with feet together
— Needs help to attain position &/or unable to hold for 30 seconds

8. Standing unsupported 1 foot in front—"Stand with 1 foot in front of the other (heel to toe)"
— Able to place feet tandem independently & hold for 30 seconds
— Able to place foot ahead of other independently & hold 30 seconds
— Able to take small step independently & hold 30 seconds or requires assistance to place foot in front but can stand for 30 seconds
— Needs help to step but can hold 15 seconds
— Loses balance while stepping or standing

(Continued text on following page)

Pediatric Balance Scale (Continued)

9. Standing on 1 leg–"Stand on 1 leg as long as able without holding on"

- Able to lift leg independently & hold 10 seconds
- Able to lift leg independently & hold 5–9 seconds
- Able to lift leg independently & hold 3–4 seconds
- Tries to lift leg; unable to hold 3 seconds but remains standing
- Unable to try or needs assist to prevent fall

10. Turn 360 degrees–"Make a full circle, STOP, & make a full circle in the other direction"

- Able to turn 360° safely in ≤ 4 seconds each way
- Able to turn 360° safely in ≤ 4 seconds in 1 direction but other direction requires > 4 seconds
- Able to turn 360° safely but slowly
- Needs close supervision or constant verbal cueing
- Needs assistance while turning

11. Turning to look behind left & right shoulder while standing still–"Stand with feet still & follow object as it is moved to each side"

- Looks over each shoulder, wt shift include trunk rotation
- Looks over 1 shoulder w/ trunk rotation, wt shift in opposite direction is to level of shoulder; no trunk rotation
- Turns head to look to level of shoulder; no trunk rotation

12. Pick up object from floor from a standing position–"Pick up object placed in front of dominant foot"

- Able to pick up object safely & easily
- Able to pick up object but needs supervision
- Unable to pick up object but reaches 1–2 inches from object & keeps balance independently
- Unable to pick up object; needs supervision while attempting

(Continued text on following page)

Pediatric Balance Scale *(Continued)*

– Needs supervision when turning; chin moves greater than 1/2 distance to shoulder
– Needs assist to keep from losing balance/falling; mov't of chin is less than 1/2 distance to shoulder

– Unable to try; needs assistance to keep from losing balance or falling

13. Placing alternate foot on step stool standing unsupported. "Place each foot alternately on the step stool & continue until eachfoot touched the stool 4 times"
– Stands independently & safely & completes 8 steps in 20 seconds
– Able to stand independently & completes 8 steps > 20 seconds
– Able to complete 4 steps w/o assistance but requires close supervision
– Able to complete 2 steps; needs minimal assistance
– Needs assistance to maintain balance or keep from falling

14. Reaching forward with outstretched arm while standing. "Stretch out your fingers, make a fist & reach forward as far as able w/o moving feet"
– Can reach forward confidently > 10 inches
– Can reach forward > 5 inches, safely
– Can reach forward > 2 inches, safely
– Reaches forward but needs supervision
– Loses balance while trying, requiring external support

Score:
Scoring: The items are scored in descending order with the top statement = 4 & the bottom statement = 0.

Maximum score = 56

Source: Franjoine MR, Gunther JS & Taylor MJ (2003).

Immunization Schedule

Vaccination	Birth	1	2	4	6	12	15	18	24	4-6
DPT			#1	#2	#3		#4			#5
OPV			#1	#2	#3					#4
MMR						#1				#2
HiB			#1	#2	#3	#4				
Hep B		#1	#2		#3					
Varicella						#1				
PCV			#1	#2	#3	#4				

DPT = Diphtheria, Pertussis, Tetanus
OPV = Oral Polio Vaccine
MMR = Measles, Mumps, Rubella
HiB = *Haemophilus influenzae* type B (meningitis)
Hep B = Hepatitis B
Varicella = Chickenpox
PCV = Pneumococcal Conjugate Vaccine

Note: These recommended ages for vaccinations are from the Dept of Health & Human Services (CDC), the Advisory Committee on Immunization Practices, the American Academy of Pediatrics, and the American Academy of Family Physicians. Any dose not given at the recommended age should be given as a "catch-up" shot at the following visit.

Contagious Childhood Diseases

RUBELLA

Contagious time & mechanism:

Most contagious 7 days before to 7 days after the rash erupts

Signs & Symptoms:

- Rash that starts on face/trunk & spreads to extremities that resolves in 3 days
- Mild fever (< 100°)
- Lymph node adenopathy
- Cough, congestion, coryza, conjunctivitis

ROSEOLA

Contagious time & mechanism:

Contagious via direct contact, cough, sneeze. Most common in children 9 months to 3 years

Signs & Symptoms:

- Beware of seizures associated with high fever
- Fever occurs 3–4 days f/b rash
- Multiple pale pink macules & papules (1–5 mm) appear on trunk & spread to extremities; may last a few hours to a few days
- Red bumps may turn white after being touched
- Cold-like symptoms

(Continued text on following page)

Contagious Childhood Diseases *(Continued)*

CHICKENPOX (Varicella)

Contagious time & mechanism:

Incubation period of 11–21 days. Contagious via droplets from cough, sneeze, or direct contact with blisters; contagious until all vesicles crust over

Signs & Symptoms

- Skin lesions–3 stages: macule, vesicle, granular scab
- Skin lesions (look like drops of water on an erythematous base) start on head/trunk & spread to limbs, buccal mucosa, scalp, axilla, URI, & conjunctiva
- Itching & general body aches
- Cold-like symptoms–fever, malaise, h/a

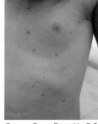

Source: From Barankin B & Freiman A (2006).

MUMPS

Contagious time & mechanism:

Contagious from 6 days prior to & up to 2 weeks after gland swelling. Spread through direct contact or airborne droplets

Signs & Symptoms:

- Enlarged salivary glands
- H/A, muscle aches, fever, difficulty swallowing (2° swelling of salivary glands), vomiting

MEASLES (Rubeloa)

Contagious time & mechanism:

Incubation time is 10–21 days. Contagious via airborne droplets or fluids in blisters from 1–2 days before blisters until they crust over

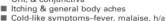

(Continued text on following page)

Contagious Childhood Diseases (Continued)

Signs & Symptoms:

- 1st signs = fever > 100°, sore throat, runny nose, cough, conjunctivitis
- Within a few days, bright red blotchy rash starts on forehead, face, neck & spreads to extremities; rash fades in 3–5 days
- Koplik's spots–small, red spots with bluish white specks in center
- Photosensitivity, otitis media, & pneumonia are 2° px

CONJUNCTIVITIS (pink eye)

Contagious time & mechanism:

Contagious via direct contact

Signs & Symptoms:

- Most common symptom is eye irritation (feels like there is a piece of sand in the eye)
- Redness & swelling of eye & eyelid
- Crust of discharge will cause eyelids to be stuck together in the morning
- Photosensitivity & itching

SCARLET FEVER

Contagious time & mechanism:

Peak prevalence is in 4–8 yr-olds. Frequently evolves from initial illness & spreads through airborne droplets.
Contagious until antibiotics are taken for 24 hrs

Signs & Symptoms:

- Fever, sore throat, h/a, & vomiting x 1–2 days f/b rash
- Pink skin rash on neck, chest, axilla, groin, & thighs
- Rash feels like sandpaper
- Strawberry tongue–initially white, then red

(Continued text on following page)

Contagious Childhood Diseases *(Continued)*

BACTERIAL MENINGITIS

Contagious time & mechanism:

Highly contagious via droplets of saliva

Signs & Symptoms:

- ■ Fever & light sensitivity
- ■ Lethargy (hypotonia) & stiff neck
- ■ Poor feeding; vomiting & headache
- ■ Respiratory distress; apnea; cyanosis
- ■ Paradoxic irritability (quiet when stationary & cries when held)
- ■ Seizures in 30–40% of cases

Source: Porth CM (1994); Boissonnault WG (2005).

Musculoskeletal Pathology

Pathology	Signs & Symptoms
Congenital torticollis	■ Chronic cervical positioning in ipsilateral SB & contralateral rotation ■ Palpable nodule in the SCM ■ Limited neck ROM ■ Skull asymmetry with side of face appearing flattened ■ As many as 1 in 5 babies with torti-collis also develop hip dysplasia ■ Strong association with reflux ■ Screen for visual tracking (CN IV)
Hip dislocation	■ May result from a breech birth or trauma ■ (+) Tests: Ortolani & Barlow ■ (+) X-ray (associated with torticollis) **Congenital** ■ Shortened limb, positioned in flexion & abduction **Posterior Traumatic (MVA)** ■ Groin & lateral hip pain ■ Shortened limb, positioned in flexion, adduction & IR **Anterior Traumatic (forced abduction)** ■ Groin pain & tenderness ■ Positioned in extension & ER if superior/anterior ■ Positioned in flexion, abduction, & ER if inferior/anterior
Legg-Calvé-Perthes Note: low birth weight (< 5.5 lb) is highly corre-lated with Legg-Calve-Perthes	■ 5–8 yo boys > girls ■ Hip, groin, &/or thigh pain resulting in antalgic gait ■ ↓ Pain with hip abduction & IR ■ (+) Trendelenburg ■ Leg length inequality; thigh atrophy

(Continued on text on following page)

Musculoskeletal Pathology *(Continued)*

Pathology	Signs & Symptoms
	■ Bone scan/MRI = early detection ■ May appear normal for several weeks, 1st sign (~4 wks) is radiolucent crescent image parallel to superior rim of femoral head ■ Need to r/o JRA & hip inflammation
Slipped capital femoral epiphysis	■ Overweight adolescent ■ Recent growth spurt ■ Groin pain with WB ■ Gradual onset of unilateral hip, thigh, & knee pain ■ Antalgic gait & ↓ limb length ■ LE held in abduction & ER (limited IR) ■ Quadriceps atrophy ■ AP x-ray needed to identify widening of physis & ↓ ht of epiphysis; lateral view = epiphyseal displacement ■ Need to r/o muscle strain & avulsion
Transient synovitis of the hip = terile effusion of unknown etiology, resolves in 2 days to 2 weeks with NSAID	■ Most common childhood hip pain ■ Age 3–10 yrs; males 2× > females ■ History of recent illness–virus, URI, bronchitis, otitis media ■ Unilateral hip/groin pain; may c/o medial thigh/groin pain with mov't ■ Child holds hip in flexion, slight abduction, & ER ■ Awakes with a limp ■ Possible low-grade fever ■ R/o septic hip, slipped capital femoral epiphysis, & Legg-Calvé-Perthes
Sever's disease (partial avulsion of calcaneal apophysis via overuse)	■ Occurs in 5–10 yo ♀ & 10–12 yo ♂ ■ Posterior heel pain ■ Swelling @ distal Achilles attachment ■ Limited dorsiflexion ■ Gait deviations

(Continued text on following page)

Musculoskeletal Pathology (Continued)

Pathology	Signs & Symptoms
Marfan syndrome (autosomal dominant inherited disorder)	■ Disproportionately long arms, leg, fingers, & toes (tall–lower body longer than upper body) ■ Kyphoscoliosis ■ Long skull with frontal prominence ■ Pectus chest (concave) ■ Slender–↑ sub-q fat ■ Weak tendons, ligaments, & jt capsules with jt hyperextensibility ■ Defective heart valves = murmur ■ High incidence of dissecting aortic aneurysm ■ Hernia ■ Sleep apnea ■ Dislocation of eye lens; myopia ■ "Thumb sign"
Ehlers-Danlos syndrome	■ Hyperextensibility of the skin ■ Score of < 5/9 on the Beighton Scale of Joint Hypermobility (see following) ■ Recurring joint dislocations ■ Bruising tendencies

Beighton Scale of Joint Hypermobility

■ Hands flat on the floor with knees straight = 1 point
■ Elbow hyperextension = 1 point each
■ Knee hyperextension = 1 point each
■ Thumb bends to touch the front of forearm = 1 point each
■ Little finger bends back 90° = 1 point each

Maximum score is 9 points

Pediatric Rheumatology Collaborative Study Group's Articular Severity Index

Rating	Swelling	Pain with Motion	Tender to Palpation	Limited Motion
0	No swelling	No pain	No tenderness	Full motion
1	Mild swelling (no loss of bony contour)	Mild pain	Mild tenderness	Limited up to 25%
2	Moderate swelling (loss of distinctive bony contour)	Withdraws limb or facial grimace with joint mov't	Withdraws limb or facial grimace with palpation	Limited up to 50%
3	Marked swelling (bulging synovial proliferation)	Responds markedly to joint mov't	Responds markedly to palpation	Limited up to 75%
4				Limited by > 75%

Source: Guzman J, Burgos-Vargas R, Duarte-Salazar C & Gomez-Mora (1995).

Muscular Dystrophy

Hereditary, progressive muscular diseases with a characteristic pattern of weakness

Duchenne	Becker's	Limb-Girdle	Facioscapu-lohumeral
■ Onset 1-5 yo	■ Onset 5-10 yo	■ Onset 10-30 yo	■ Onset 1st decade
■ Rarely dx before age 3	■ A similar presentation of a less severe form than Duchenne's	■ Muscles of shoulders & hips are affected 1st	■ Muscles of shoulders & face are affected
■ Rapidly progressing muscle weakness LE > UE	■ Slow onset of muscle weakness LE > UE	■ Waddling gait	■ Expressionless appearance
■ Frequent falls, waddling gait, poor balance	■ Frequent falls, waddling gait, poor balance	■ Difficulty rising from sitting, reaching over-head, & carrying heavy objects	■ Large variations in muscle weakness
■ Difficulty with stairs, running, hopping, jumping	■ Difficulty with stairs, running, hopping, jumping	■ Pain usually not a factor	■ Weakness can be asymmetrical
■ Enlarged calf muscles (pseudohypertrophy)	■ Enlarged calf muscles	■ Prognosis–progressive loss of function over 20-30 yrs; WC needed for mobility & end-stage respiratory compromise	■ Winged scapula
■ Toe walking	■ Lordosis, scoliosis		■ Pain usually not a factor
■ Lordosis, scoliosis	■ Pain usually not a factor		■ Prognosis–slower progression & lesser loss of function; normal life span
■ Fatigue	■ Fatigue		
■ Pain usually not a factor	■ Prognosis–slower progression than Duchenne's; may continue walking into adulthood		
■ Average IQ = 85			
■ Prognosis–braces to ambulate, WC use @ puberty, life span < 25 yrs (end-stage respiratory px)			

Neuromuscular Pathology

Possible Red Flags for Autism, Pervasive Dev't Disorder, or Communication Disorders:

■ Child does not respond to his/her name	Yes	No
■ Child cannot explain what he/she wants	Yes	No
■ Language skills or speech are delayed	Yes	No
■ Child doesn't follow directions	Yes	No
■ At times, the child seems to be deaf	Yes	No
■ Child seems to hear sometimes, but not others	Yes	No
■ Child doesn't point or wave bye-bye	Yes	No
■ Child used to say a few words or babble, but now he/she doesn't	Yes	No
■ Child throws intense or violent tantrums	Yes	No
■ Child has odd movement patterns	Yes	No
■ Child is hyperactive, uncooperative, or oppositional	Yes	No
■ Child doesn't know how to play with toy	Yes	No
■ Child seems to prefer to play alone	Yes	No
■ Child doesn't smile when smiled at	Yes	No
■ Child has poor eye contact	Yes	No
■ Child gets "stuck" on things over & over & can't move on to other things	Yes	No
■ Child gets things for him/herself only	Yes	No
■ Child is very independent for his/her age	Yes	No
■ Child does things "early" compared to other children	Yes	No
■ Child seems to be in his/her "own world"	Yes	No
■ Child seems to tune people out	Yes	No
■ Child is not interested in other children	Yes	No
■ Child walks on his/her toes	Yes	No
■ Child shows unusual attachments to toys, objects, or schedules	Yes	No
■ Child spends a lot of time lining things up	Yes	No

Source: "Autism Facts" by the National Institute of Child Health & Human Development.

Signs & Symptoms of Autism & Pervasive Dev't Disorder (PDD)

Autism = 6 of 12 symptoms across 3 areas & PDD = < 6 of 12 symptoms

Communication	Social Interactions	Behavior
■ Delay in, or total lack of, development of spoken language ■ Difficulty initiating conversation ■ Echolalia (repeating words or phrases instead of using normal language) ■ Does not respond to name ■ Does not use or respond to gestures and other nonverbal cues	■ Does not point to objects or show them to others ■ Does not make eye contact at appropriate times ■ Does not look at other people's faces as much ■ Does not respond to facial expressions or body language ■ Does not smile back at others ■ Lack of peer relationships appropriate to age level ■ Less interest in other children ■ Not motivated by praise or physical affection ■ Does not clearly demonstrate sympathy or empathy	■ Engages in highly repetitive play ■ Obsessively preoccupied with a specific interest or object ■ Lack of make-believe or imitative play ■ Dependent on routines, rituals, and familiarity ■ Repetitive body mov'ts (hand or finger flapping, eye rolling, twisting, spinning, rocking, etc.) ■ Preoccupation with parts of objects ■ Easily overstimulated by noises, crowds, or lights ■ Extreme dislike of certain sounds, textures, or situations ■ Does not have strong response to pain

Possible Signs & Symptoms in a Child with Asperger Syndrome (AS)

- Inappropriate or minimal social interactions
- Conversations almost always revolving around self rather than others
- "Scripted," "robotic," or repetitive speech
- Lack of "common sense"
- Problems with reading, math, or writing skills
- Obsession with complex topics such as patterns or music
- Average to above-average verbal cognitive abilities
- Average to below-average nonverbal cognitive abilities
- Awkward movements
- Odd behaviors or mannerisms

Note: Acquisition of language milestones are on time. It's not uncommon for a child to be diagnosed with attention-deficit hyperactivity disorder (ADHD) before the diagnosis of AS is made later on.

Signs & Symptoms of ADHD

By definition, behavior must appear before age 7 & persist for 6 months & disrupt 2 of the following—home, school, work, or social environments

- Inattention = easily distracted, forgetful, can't seem to get or stay focused, does not appear to listen
- Hyperactivity = trouble staying still, fidgeting, squirming, restless, difficulty awaiting one's turn, interrupting, excessive talking
- Impulsivity = often acts without thinking, unable to control impulses

Source: http://www.adhdhelp.net/

Signs & Symptoms of Lead Poisoning

- Peripheral motor neuropathy
  - Radial nerve = wrist drop
  - Peroneal nerve = foot drop
- GI pain
- Anemia
- Intellectual/motor deficits
- Renal tubular acidosis
- Lead line of the gingival/gums

Tourette's Syndrome

Defined by multiple motor & vocal tics lasting for > 1 year

- Becomes evident between 2 and 15 years of age
- Most common 1st symptom is a facial tic (eye blink, nose twitch, grimace)
- Involuntary movements (tics) of the arms, limbs, or trunk
- Other symptoms, such as touching, repetitive thoughts & movements & compulsions, can occur
- Verbal tics (vocalizations) usually occur with the mov'ts
- Although unusual, verbal tics may also be expressed as coprolalia (the involuntary use of obscene words) or copropraxia (obscene gestures)

Source: http://www.tsa-usa.org/aboutts.html.

Down Syndrome

- Mental retardation
- Flat facial features
- Low/flat bridged nose
- Epicanthal folds of eyes (oriental appearance, hence mongoloid)
- Enlarged ears
- Prominent tongue
- Joint hypermobility
- Congenital cardiac disease (septal defects, ductus arteriosus)
- Short stature
- Simian crease (single transverse crease across palm)
- Broad hands & feet with short fingers & toes
- Short neck, small head, small oral cavity
- GI malformation
- Possible sterility
- ↑ Risk of leukemia (< 15 yo)

Possible Signs & Symptoms of a Brain Tumor

- H/A–↑ intracranial pressure
- Vomiting
- Visual changes
- Mentation changes
- Seizures
- Muscle weakness
- Bladder dysfunction
- Coordination changes
- (+) Babinski
- Clonus (ankle or wrist)

Fetal Alcohol Syndrome (FAS)

Physical Features

Discriminating Features

Secondary Features

- Small eye slits
- Flat midface
- Short nose
- Indistinct philtrum
- Trim upper lip
- Epicanthal folds
- Low nasal bridge
- Minor ear anomalies
- Pointed chin

Source: Effgen, S (2005).

Cognitive Concerns

- Attention deficit disorder
- Hyperactivity
- Learning disabilities
- Memory problems & intellectual impairment
- Delayed development
- Attachment issues
- Neurosensory hearing loss
- Impaired visual/spatial skills
- Problems with reasoning & judgment
- Inability to appreciate consequences
- Behavioral issues

Source: National Organization on Fetal Alcohol Syndrome (http:www.nofas.org).

Cardiovascular & Pulmonary Pathology

Normal Predicted Average Peak Expiratory Flow (L/min) Normal Children & Adolescents

Height (inches)	Peak Expiratory Flow	Height (inches)	Peak Expiratory Flow
43	147	55	307
44	160	56	320
45	173	57	334
46	187	58	347
47	200	59	360
48	214	60	373
49	227	61	387
50	240	62	400
51	254	63	413
52	267	64	427
53	280	65	440
54	293	66	454

Asthma attack: Failure to experience a 15% increase in Peak Expiratory Flow after 2 puffs of an inhaler within 5 minutes, consider emergency care.

Source: Nunn I & Gregg AJ (1973).

Asthma

Triggers

- Respiratory infections
- Exercise
- Cigarette smoke
- Cold environments
- Stress
- Allergic reactions
- Pollutants

Signs & Symptoms

- Wheezing
- Prolonged expiration
- Difficulty breathing
- Cough
- SOB

Asthma Inhalers

- **Short-acting bronchodilator** = immediate symptom relief; e.g., albuterol (Proventil, Ventolin), pirbuterol (Maxair)
- **Long-acting bronchodilators** = up to 12 hrs of symptom relief; e.g., salmeterol (Serevent); formoterol (Foradil)
- **Corticosteroids** = long-term prevention of symptoms, may take up to 7 days for peak effectiveness; e.g., beclomethasone dipropionate (QVAR); fluticasone (Flovent); budesonide (Pulmicort); triamcinolone acetonide (Azmacort);flunisolide (AeroBid)
- **Nonsteroidals** = long-term prevention of inflammation; e.g., Cromolyn, nedocromil
- **Corticosteroid + bronchodilator** = long-acting combination; e.g., Advair

Complications of Cystic Fibrosis (can vary greatly)	
Lung Complications	**GI Complications**
■ Persistent cough, excessive phlegm ■ Wheezing, short of breath ■ Frequent lung infections, e.g., pneumonia, bronchitis ■ Chronic bronchiectasis ■ Chronic sinusitis or asthma ■ Progressive lung deterioration	■ Poor absorption of nutrients ■ Large appetite with poor weight gain ■ Poor growth ■ Greasy, thick stools ■ Chronic pancreatitis ■ Meconium ileus (obstructed intestine in newborns)

Note: More than 90% of cystic fibrosis patients have saltier sweat than people without the disease. One of the diagnostic tests measures the amount of salt in the sweat.

Integumentary Pathology

CONTACT DERMATITIS–POISON IVY

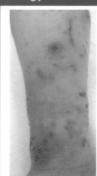

■ The rash itself is not contagious, & fluid in blisters does not spread rash. Poison ivy dermatitis appears 4 hours to 10 days after exposure, depending on individual sensitivity & the amount of exposure.

■ The rash is self-limited; & will clear up without treatment. Letting nature take its course with mild poison ivy dermatitis is reasonable, but severe rashes need treatment to ease the misery & disability they cause. First time with a rash takes longer to clear up than a repeat attack (~3–4 weeks).

Source: From Barankin B & Freiman A (2006).

(Continued text on following page)

Integumentary Pathology (Continued)

IMPETIGO-Bacterial

- Peak prevalence is in preschool children
- Contagious via direct contact with infected area
- Usually occurs around nose & mouth
- Characterized by thin-walled blisters that burst, rupture, ooze fluid, & develop a yellow-crusted lesion
- Scratching can spread infection

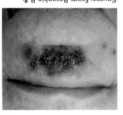

Source: From Barankin B & Freiman A (2006).

RINGWORM

- Fungal infection
- Contagious via skin contact with infected person/pet or with an object the infected person touched
- Rash appears 4–14 days after contact
- Ring-sized blotch (1/2–1" diameter)
- Scaly with clear center
- May be itchy
- Body builds a natural immunity in ~15 wks, but antifungal cream resolves rash faster.

(Continued text on following page)

Integumentary Pathology *(Continued)*

VIRAL WARTS

- Benign cutaneous tumors 2° HPV
- Primary locations = hands, feet, face, genitals
- Dome-shaped nodules with dark spots (thrombosed capillaries)

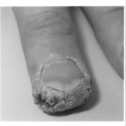

Source: From Barankin B & Freiman A (2006).

HERPES SIMPLEX

- Common vesicular eruptions that are highly contagious & spread by direct contact
- Vesicles are painful & the mucous membranes erode quickly
- Other symptoms = fever, malaise, swollen lymph nodes (not to be confused with impetigo)

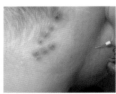

Source: From Barankin B & Freiman A (2006).

LATEX ALLERGY

- Onset can be within minutes or over a few days
- Erythema, vesicles, papules, pruritus, blisters, crusting
- Hives (urticaria), faintness, nausea, vomiting, abdominal cramps, rhinoconjunctivitis, bronchospasm, anaphylactic shock

Lyme Disease

Note: This is a multisystemic inflammatory condition. The transmission of the tick spirochete takes ~ 48 hrs. Blood work is used to confirm the disease, not to diagnose it. Clinician should r/o GBS, MS, & FMS.

Early Localized Stage

- Rash & onset of erythema in 7–14 days (range = 3–30 days)
- Rash may be solid red expanding rash or a central spot with rings (bull's-eye)
- Average diameter of rash is 5–6"
- Rash may or may not be warm to palpation
- Rash is usually not painful or itchy
- Fever
- Malaise
- Headache
- Muscle aches; joint pain

Early Disseminated Stage

- ≥ 2 rashes not @ the bite site
- Migrating pain
- Headache; stiff neck; facial palsy
- Numbness/tingling into extremities
- Abnormal pulse
- Sore throat
- Visual changes
- 100–102° fever
- Severe fatigue

Late Stage

- Arthritis of 1–2 larger joints
- Neurological changes–disorientation, confusion, dizziness, mental "fog," numbness in extremities
- Visual impairment
- Cardiac irregularities

Source: American Lyme Disease Foundation.

Gastrointestinal Pathology

Infantile Colic

Defined as 3 hrs of arbitrary crying/day, 3 days/wk for 3 wks

- Generally occurs from 2 weeks to 4–5 months
- May be related to intestinal intolerance of cow's milk
- Associated with face flushing, pulling knees to chest, passing gas, difficulty having bowel mov'ts

Reflux

At least 50% of infants have some level of reflux for the few couple of months of life; if >1 of the following signs/symptoms persist after several months, a consultation for Infantile Reflux or GERD should be considered:

- Refusing food or accepting only a few bites despite being hungry
- Requiring constant small meals or liquid
- Food/oral aversions
- Anemia
- Excessive drooling
- Running nose, sinus or ear infections
- Swallowing problems, gagging, choking
- Chronic hoarse voice
- Frequent red, sore throat without infection present
- Apnea
- Respiratory problems—pneumonia, bronchitis, wheezing, asthma, night-time cough, aspiration
- Poor weight gain, weight loss, failure to thrive
- Erosion of dental enamel & bad breath
- Neck arching (Sandifer's syndrome)

Infant Reflux Impact Survey		
Does your child take a daily medication for his/her reflux, other than antacids, that do not appear to be helping the symptoms?	Yes	No
Does your child's reflux interfere with his/her activities, quality of life, or playtime?	Yes	No
Has mealtime become a battle ground?	Yes	No
Is your child's throwing up causing weight loss and health issues?	Yes	No
Do the symptoms persist even after changing formula or diet changes if you are breastfeeding?	Yes	No
Is the child's sleep interrupted frequently?	Yes	No
Is your baby having difficulty gaining or sustaining sufficient weight?	Yes	No
Does your child suffer from frequent ear, sinus or respiratory infections, sound hoarse, or have difficulty breathing?	Yes	No
Does baby or child appear to be miserable or in pain most of, or a large part of the day, particularly after mealtime?	Yes	No
Does your child's reflux not seem to improve despite maximum efforts at all the lifestyle modifications mentioned?	Yes	No

Source: http://www.infantrefluxdisease.com/

Appendicitis

Mean age for appendicitis in children is 6–10 yrs old

Signs & Symptoms–in order of significant likelihood ratios	Differential Diagnosis
■ Ⓡ LQ pain, (+) McBurney's point → Ⓡ thigh/testicle ■ Nausea, vomiting, night sweats ■ Guarding of rectus abdominis ■ (+) Psoas sign ■ (+) Obturator sign ■ Low-grade fever unless associated with perforation (then high fever may occur) ■ (+) Rebound tenderness ■ Position of relief: tense abdomen with FB or lie down with both knees to chest	■ ↓ Hemoglobin ■ ↓ Hematocrit ■ Change in fingernail beds ■ Pale skin color ■ Fatigue ■ ↓ DBP

Source: American Family Physician
http://www.afp.org/afp/991101ap/2027.html.

Hepatic Pathology

Signs & Symptoms of Baby Jaundice

■ Yellowing of the skin & whites of the eyes
■ Pale & "fatty" texture to stool (stools in newborns should be green/yellow)
■ Yellow urine (urine in newborns should be colorless)

Note: If jaundice continues beyond 14 days of age for a full-term baby or 21 days in a premature baby, then this should be investigated.

Endocrine Pathology

Signs & Symptoms of Type 1 (Juvenile) Diabetes

- High levels of sugar in blood
- High levels of sugar in urine
- Frequent urination in larger volumes (kidney trying to flush excess glucose)
- Abnormally thirsty (attempts to replace fluid loss)
- Extreme hunger but loses weight
- Blurred vision
- Fatigue, irritability, & mood changes (no glucose for energy)
- Abdominal pain, nausea, vomiting, & fruity-smelling breath (build-up of ketones)
- Onset of bedwetting in a child with no prior px
- Vaginal yeast infection in ♀ prior to puberty

Urogenital Pathology

Signs & Symptoms of a Urinary Tract Infection in a Child

- Dysuria
- Frequency
- Malodorous urine
- Dribbling/hesitancy
- Hematuria
- Squatting
- Enuresis (when toilet trained)
- Suprapubic-flank pain
- Fever

Source: Ahmed SM & Swedlund SK (1998).

Other Pathology

Pediatric Malignancies

- **Ewing's sarcoma**
  - Rare type of bone cancer–localized or metastatic
  - Peak incidence is 10–20 years old
  - 1° locations = pelvis, thigh, lower leg, upper arm, & rib
  - Pathologic fx are rare
  - 1st symptom is intermittent but intense pain
  - Remittent fever, mild anemia, wt loss
  - Eventually a large palpable mass
- **Lymphoma (Hodgkin's disease)**
  - Rare in children < 5 yo; more common in ♂ from 5–10 yrs
  - Painless swelling of lymph nodes in neck or axilla
  - Fever & night sweats
  - Weight loss
- **Leukemia**
  - Difficult to diagnose because of the similarity to normal childhood diseases
  - Onset can be slow or rapid
  - Fever & loss of appetite
  - Pale skin & frequent bruising
  - Enlarged cervical lymph nodes
  - Abdominal protrusion 2° enlargement of spleen & liver
  - ↑ Irritability
- **Neuroblastoma**
  - Most common solid tumor of children under 5 yrs
  - Originates in sympathetic nervous tissue
  - Most common site is abdomen (near adrenal gland)
  - 1st signs are fatigue & loss of appetite
  - Abdominal swelling may result in constipation, px with urination, & breathlessness
- **Pilocytic astrocytoma (peaks at 5–14 yo)**
  - H/A–worse in AM
  - H/A ↑ with activity, Valsalva, stooping (↑ intracranial pressure)
  - Seizures
  - Visual changes
  - Vomiting
  - Ataxia

Growth & Development

NOTE: See Pediatric Tab for height & weight charts.

Age Yr	BP % -tile	SBP (mm Hg) for Boys			DBP (mm Hg) for Boys		
		Percentile of Height			Percentile of Height		
		5th	50th	95th	5th	50th	95th
10	50th	97	102	106	58	61	63
	95th	115	119	123	77	80	82
11	50th	99	104	107	59	61	63
	95th	117	121	125	78	80	82
12	50th	101	106	110	59	62	64
	95th	119	123	127	78	81	83
13	50th	104	108	112	60	62	64
	95th	121	126	130	79	81	83
14	50th	106	111	115	60	63	65
	95th	124	128	132	80	82	84
15	50th	109	113	117	61	64	66
	95th	126	131	135	81	83	85
16	50th	111	116	120	63	65	67
	95th	129	134	137	82	84	87
17	50th	114	118	122	65	67	70
	95th	131	136	140	84	87	89

Growth & Development (Continued)

Age Yr	BP % -tile	SBP (mm Hg) for Girls			DBP (mm Hg) for Girls		
		Percentile of Height			Percentile of Height		
		5th	50th	95th	5th	50th	95th
10	50th	98	102	105	59	60	62
	95th	116	119	122	77	78	80
11	50th	100	103	107	60	61	63
	95th	118	121	124	78	79	81
12	50th	102	105	109	61	62	64
	95th	119	123	126	79	80	82
13	50th	104	107	110	62	63	65
	95th	121	124	135	80	81	83
14	50th	106	109	112	63	64	66
	95th	123	126	129	81	82	84
15	50th	107	110	113	64	65	67
	95th	124	123	131	82	83	85
16	50th	108	111	114	64	66	68
	95th	125	128	132	82	84	86
17	50th	108	111	115	64	66	68
	95th	125	129	132	82	84	86

Musculoskeletal Pathology

Pathology	Signs & Symptoms
Osgood-Schlatter syndrome	■ Occurs in 10–15 yo ♂ & 10–11 yo ♀ ■ Intermittent aching pain at tibial tubercle & distal patellar tendon ■ Enlarged tibial tuberosity ■ Tight quads & hamstrings resulting in ↑ AROM ■ Effusion results in knee extensor lag ■ (+) Ely test (tight rectus femoris) ■ (+) X-ray for avulsion of tibial tuberosity (lateral view) ■ Need to r/o avascular necrosis
Sinding-Larsen-Johansson syndrome	■ Partial avulsion of inferior pole of patella in 10–15 yo ♂ ■ Anterior knee pain & TTP at distal pole of the patella with knee extension ■ Antalgic gait ■ ↑ Knee ROM ■ X-ray (lateral view) = fragmentation of inferior patella pole
Slipped capital femoral epiphysis **Note:** occurs in boys 2× > girls; higher incidence in African American population; ↑ incidence with growth hormone deficiency	■ Overweight adolescent ■ Recent growth spurt ■ Gradual onset of unilateral hip, thigh, & knee pain ■ Groin pain with WB ■ Antalgic gait & ↓ limb length ■ LE held in ER & abduction with ■ Hip goes into ER (limited IR) ■ Passive hip flexion ■ Quadriceps atrophy ■ AP x-ray needed to identify widening of physis & ↑ ht of epiphysis; lateral view = epiphyseal displacement ■ Need to r/o muscle strain & avulsion

(Continued text on following page)

Musculoskeletal Pathology (Continued)

Pathology	Signs & Symptoms
Compartment syndrome **Beware:** This is an emergency situation	■ Soft tissue pressures via fluid accumulation ■ Ischemia of extensor hallucis longus ■ Skin feels warm & firm ■ Pain with stretch or AROM; foot drop ■ Most reliable sign is sensory deficit of dorsum of foot in 1st interdigital cleft ■ Pulses are normal until the end & then surgery within 4–6 hours is required to prevent muscle necrosis & nerve damage ■ Confirmed with MRI & pressure assessment
Marfan syndrome	■ Disproportionately long arms, leg, fingers, & toes (tall–lower body longer than upper body) ■ Long skull with frontal prominence ■ Kyphoscoliosis ■ Pectus chest (concave) ■ Slender–↓ sub-q fat ■ Weak tendons, ligaments, & joint capsules with joint hyperextensibility ■ Defective heart valves = murmur ■ High incidence of dissecting aortic aneurysm ■ Hernia ■ Sleep apnea ■ Dislocation of eye lens; myopia ■ "Thumb sign"

Pediatric Rheumatology Collaborative Study Group's Articular Severity Index

Rating	Swelling	Pain with Motion	Tender to Palpation	Limited Motion
0	No swelling	No pain	No tenderness	Full motion
1	Mild swelling (no loss of bony contour)	Mild pain	Mild tenderness	Limited up to 25%
2	Moderate swelling (loss of distinctive bony contour)	Withdraws limb or facial grimace with jt mov't	Withdraws limb or facial grimace with palpation	Limited up to 50%
3	Marked swelling (bulging synovial proliferation)	Responds markedly to jt mov't	Responds markedly to palpation	Limited up to 75%
4				Limited by > 75%

Source: Guzman J, Burgos-Vargas R, Duarte-Salazar C & Gomez-Mora (1995).

Signs & Symptoms of Anabolic Steroid Abuse

- Anxiety & chest pain
- ↓ HDL & ↑ LDL
- ↑ BP
- ↑ Weight gain in short period of time (10–15 lbs in 2–3 wks)
- Acne on face, chest, & upper back
- Needle marks
- Frequent hematomas
- Peripheral edema
- Rapid mood swings & sudden anger ("Roid Rage")
- Growth plate closure
- Jaundice
- Alopecia
- Tumors & cancer
- Females: abnormal body hair, deeper voice, irregular menstruation
- Males: gynecomastia

Ottawa Knee Rules

X-ray series of the *knee* is only required if the patient presents with any of the following criteria:

- \> 55 years old
- Isolated tenderness of the patella
- Tenderness of the head of the fibula
- Inability to flex > 90 degrees
- Inability to bear weight (4 steps) *both* immediately after injury & in emergency department (regardless of limping)

Ottawa Ankle Rules

X-ray series of the *ankle* is only required if the patient presents with any of the following criteria:

- Bone tenderness at posterior edge of the distal 6 cm of the medial malleolus
- Bone tenderness at posterior edge of the distal 6 cm of the lateral malleolus
- Totally unable to bear weight *both* immediately after injury & (for 4 steps) in the emergency department

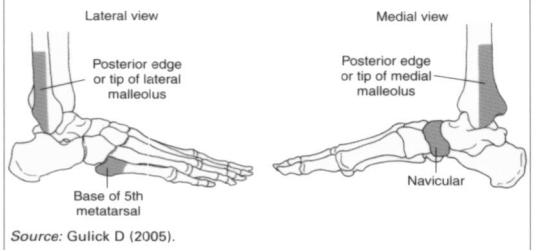

Lateral view

Posterior edge or tip of lateral malleolus

Base of 5th metatarsal

Medial view

Posterior edge or tip of medial malleolus

Navicular

Source: Gulick D (2005).

Ottawa Foot Rules

X-ray series of the *foot* is only required if the patient presents with any of the following criteria:

- Bone tenderness at navicular
- Bone tenderness at the base of 5th MT
- Totally unable to bear weight *both* immediately after injury & (for 4 steps) in the emergency department

Neuromuscular Pathology

Torg Concussion Classifications

	Grade 1	Grade 2	Grade 3	Grade 4	Grade 5
LOC	No	No	No	Yes < 5 min	Yes > 5 min
Confusion	None	Slight	Moderate	Severe	Severe
Amnesia	No	< 30 min post-traumatic amnesia	Retrograde & < 30 min post-traumatic amnesia	Retrograde & > 30 min post-traumatic amnesia	Retrograde & > 24 hrs post-traumatic amnesia
Residual symptoms	No	Perhaps	Sometimes	Yes	Yes
Dizziness	No	Mild	Moderate	Severe	Usually severe
Tinnitus	No	Mild	Moderate	Severe	Often severe
Headache	No	May be dull	Often	Often	Often
Disorientation & unsteadiness	Minimal if any	Some	Moderate	Severe (5–10 min)	Often severe (> 10 min)
Blurred vision	No	No	No	Not usually	Possible
Personality changes	No	No	No	Possible	Possible

Source: Vegso IJ & Torg JS (1991).

Systemic Lupus Erythematosus

An autoimmune disease of unknown etiology that results in:

- Inflammation & damage to various organs
- Onset: 15-45 yo; ♀ > ♂ 10-15:1
- African (3× more common), Native American, Asian > Caucasian

Signs & Symptoms

- Unexplained fever
- Swollen glands
- Photosensitivity
- Unusual hair loss
- Pale or purple fingers or toes from cold or stress (Raynaud's phenomenon)
- CNS px–seizures, h/a, periph- eral neuropathy, CVA, OBS
- Mouth, nose, vaginal ulcers
- Symptoms get worse during menstruation

- Constitutional symptoms
- Arthralgia–symmetrical
- Swollen joints
- Skin rash–"butterfly" pattern (cheeks)
- Chest pain upon deep breathing
- Extreme fatigue

Complications of Lupus

- Seizures/psychosis
- Anemia
- Pleuritis/pericarditis
- Endocarditis/myocarditis
- Glomerulonephritis

Note: A severe side effect of the acne medication minocycline is lupus-like symptoms.

Tourette's Syndrome

Defined by multiple motor & vocal tics lasting for > 1 year

- Becomes evident between 2 and 15 years of age
- Most common 1st symptom is a facial tic (eye blink, nose twitch, grimace)
- Involuntary movements (tics) of the arms, limbs, or trunk
- Other symptoms, such as touching, repetitive thoughts & movements, & compulsions, can occur
- Verbal tics (vocalizations) usually occur with the mov'ts
- Although unusual, verbal tics may also be expressed as coprolalia (the involuntary use of obscene words) or copropraxia (obscene gestures)

Source: http://www.tsa-usa.org/aboutts.html.

Possible Signs & Symptoms of a Brain Tumor

- H/A–↑ intracranial pressure
- Vomiting
- Visual changes
- Mentation changes
- Seizures
- Muscle weakness
- Bladder dysfunction
- Coordination changes
- (+) Babinski
- Clonus (ankle or wrist)

Cardiovascular & Pulmonary Pathology

Risk Factors for Development of Coronary Artery Disease

- Cigarette smoking
- High cholesterol
- Hypertension
- Obesity
- Physical inactivity
- Diabetes
- Oral contraceptives
- Alcohol consumption

Anemia

Causes

- Chemotherapy
- AIDS
- GI bleed
- RA
- CA
- Surgery
- Lupus

Signs & Symptoms

- Hemoglobin ↑
- Hematocrit ↑
- Change in fingernail beds
- Pale skin color
- Fatigue
- ↑ DBP

Source: Goodman C & Snyder T (2000).

Asthma

Triggers

- Respiratory infections
- Exercise
- Cold environments
- Cigarette smoke
- Stress
- Allergic reactions
- Pollutants

Signs & Symptoms

- Wheezing
- Cough
- Prolonged expiration
- SOB
- Difficulty breathing

Asthma Inhalers

- **Short-acting bronchodilator** = immediate symptom relief; e.g., albuterol (Proventil, Ventolin), pirbuterol (Maxair)
- **Long-acting bronchodilators** = up to 12 hrs of symptom relief; e.g., salmeterol (Serevent); formoterol (Foradil)
- **Corticosteroids** = long-term prevention of symptoms; may take up to 7 days for peak effectiveness; e.g., beclomethasone dipropionate (QVAR); fluticasone (Flovent); budesonide (Pulmicort); triamcinolone acetonide (Azmacort); flunisolide (AeroBid)
- **Nonsteroidals** = long-term prevention of inflammation; e.g., Cromolyn, nedocromil
- **Corticosteroid** + **bronchodilator** = long-acting combination; e.g., Advair

Normal Predicted Average Peak Expiratory Flow (L/min)

Normal Children & Adolescents

Height (inches)	Peak Expiratory Flow	Height (inches)	Peak Expiratory Flow
43	147	55	307
44	.160	56	320
45	173	57	334
46	187	58	347
47	200	59	360
48	214	60	373
49	227	61	387
50	240	62	400
51	254	63	413
52	267	64	427
53	280	65	440
54	293	66	454

Asthma attack: Failure to experience a 15% increase in Peak Expiratory Flow after 2 puffs of an inhaler within 5 minutes, consider emergency care.

Source: Nunn I & Gregg AJ (1973).

Integumentary Pathology

FOLLICULITIS

- Damage to a hair follicle due to friction, blockage, or shaving
- Painful hair follicle infection with papules
- Enlarged lymph nodes
- May be contagious

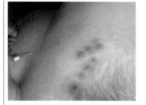

Source: From Barankin B & Freiman A (2006).

FEVER BLISTERS (HERPES SIMPLEX-TYPE 1)

- Clusters of small, clear blisters
- Appear on lips & face

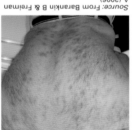

Source: From Barankin B & Freiman A (2006).

(Continued text on following page)

Integumentary Pathology *(Continued)*

CONTACT DERMATITIS–POISON IVY

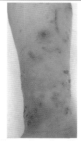

- The rash itself is not contagious, & fluid in the blisters does not spread rash. Poison ivy dermatitis appears as soon 4 hours to 10 days after the exposure, depending on sensitivity & the amount of exposure.
- The rash is self-limited & will clear up without treatment. Letting nature take its course with mild poison ivy dermatitis is reasonable, but severe rashes need treatment to ease the misery & disability they cause. First time with a rash takes longer to clear up than a repeat attack (~3–4 weeks).

Source: From Barankin B & Freiman A (2006).

RINGWORM

- Fungal infection
- Contagious via skin contact with infected person/pet or with an object the infected person touched.
- Rash appear days after contact
- Ring- or coin-sized blotch (1/2–1" diameter)
- Scaly with clear center
- May be itchy
- Body builds a natural immunity in ~15 weeks, but antifungal cream resolves rash faster

VIRAL WARTS

- Benign cutaneous tumors 2° HPV
- Primary locations = hands, feet, face, genitals
- Dome-shaped nodules with dark spots (thrombosed capillaries)

Source: From Barankin B & Freiman A (2006).

Gastrointestinal Pathology

Ulcers

- Hx of NSAID use or presence of *H. pylori* infection
- Dull gnawing/burning into midline T6–12 & radiating suprascapula
- Antacids provide temporary relief
- Nausea, coffee-grounds vomitus
- Bloody or black-tarry stools (melena)
- May have weeks of remission

Gastric	Duodenal
30–60 min after a meal	2–3 hrs after a meal
Epigastric cramping	
Localized tenderness	
Ⓛ UQ	Ⓡ of midline

Appendicitis

Onset: Most common in adolescents and young adults

Signs & Symptoms—in order of significant likelihood ratios	Differential Diagnosis
- Ⓡ LQ pain; (+) McBurney's point; pain into Ⓡ thigh/testicle - Nausea, vomiting, night sweats - Guarding of rectus abdominis - (+) Psoas sign - (+) Obturator sign - Low-grade fever - (+) Rebound tenderness - Position of relief: tense abdomen with FB or lie down with both knees to chest	- ↑ Hemoglobin - ↑ Hematocrit - Change in fingernail beds - Pale skin color - Fatigue - ↑ DBP

Source: American Family Physician
http://www.afp.org/afp/991101ap/2027.html

Bowel Pathology

Inflammatory Bowel (Crohn's or Ulcerative Colitis)	Irritable Bowel	Colon/Rectal Cancer
■ Joint arthralgia ■ Skin lesions (ankles, shins) ■ Light sensitivity ■ ↓ Pain with gas/ BM ■ Anemia due to blood loss ■ Wt loss ■ Clubbing of fingers ■ Fever ■ Rectal bleeding ■ (+) Psoas test	■ Affects females in early adulthood ■ Stress related ■ Variable/ intermittent S&S ■ Abdominal cramps ■ Nausea & vomiting ■ Flatulence ■ Change in bowel patterns ■ Foul breath	■ Hemorrhoids ■ Rectal bleeding ■ Back pain referred to LEs ■ Change in bowel patterns ■ Nausea & vomiting ■ Wt loss ■ Fatigue & dyspnea due to iron deficiency ■ Red/mahogany stools

Hepatic Pathology

Epstein-Barr Virus (Mononucleosis)

Symptom TRIAD (lasts 1–4 wks)

■ Fever	■ Sore throat	■ Swollen lymph glands

Associated Signs & Symptoms

■ ↑ WBC & lymphocytes ■ (+) Reaction to "Mono Spot" test	■ (+) Paul-Bunnell heterophil antibody test ■ Swollen spleen ■ Liver px

Endocrine Pathology

Signs & Symptoms of Diabetes

- Fatigue, lethargy
- Wt loss
- Paresthesia (feet & hands)
- ↓ Urination
- ↑ Thirst
- ↑ Hunger

Abnormal Blood Glucose

Hypoglycemia

- Blood glucose < 50–60 mg/dL
- Skin is pale, cool, diaphoretic
- Disoriented or agitated
- Headache
- Blurred vision
- Slurred speech
- Tachycardia/palpitations
- Weak/shaky/LOC
- Lip/tongue numbness

Hyperglycemia

- Blood glucose > 180 mg/dL
- Skin is dry & flushed
- Fruity breath odor
- Blurred vision
- Dizziness
- Weakness
- Nausea
- Vomiting
- Cramping
- Increased urination
- LOC/seizure

Urogenital Pathology

Risks of Oral Contraceptives

- Retinal artery thrombosis
- CVA
- Pulmonary emboli
- MI
- Hepatic vein thrombosis
- Mesenteric thrombosis
- Thrombophlebitis
- Jaundice
- Hepatic adenoma
- Gallstones

Source: Rubin E & Faber JL (1994).

Endometriosis

Part of the spectrum of Pelvic Inflammatory Disease (PID)

- 30–40 yo
- Worse premenstrually & during menses
- Pain with intercourse
- Recurrent lumbosacral pain
- Infertility

Cystitis-Pyelonephritis (UTI)

- Pain with micturition
- Leukocytes & bacteria in urine (white casts)
- Cloudy urine
- Back pain
- Fever, chills
- Nausea
- Loss of appetite
- Pain with percussion over kidneys

Ectopic Pregnancy

Risk Factors

- History of pelvic inflammatory disease
- Endometriosis
- History of pelvic surgery
- Previous history of ectopic pregnancy

Signs & Symptoms

- Lower abdominal pain
- Pelvic or LB pain
- Pain referring into the shoulder girdle
- Rebound tenderness

Note: Fallopian tube will typically rupture by the 12th week of pregnancy.

Testicular Torsion

- Most common 8–30 yo
- Severe distress
- Nausea, vomiting
- Tachycardia
- Testis is large/tender with pain radiating to inguinal area
- Testicle is high in scrotum

Sexually Transmitted Diseases (STD)

Genital Herpes

- Tingling, itching, genital pain
- Eruption of small pustules & vesicles
- Lesion rupture @ ~5 day to wet ulcers
- Dysuria & urine retention
- Fever, h/a, malaise, muscle ache, lymphadenopathy

Candidiasis = yeast infection, thrush

- Results from antibiotic therapy, ↓ hormone levels (pregnancy), oral contraceptives), DM

Gonorrhea

Transmitted via sexual intercourse or from mom to infant at birth (3–5 day incubation period)

- Urethral pain, dysuria
- Dyspareunia
- Discharge
- Vaginal bleeding (unusual or after intercourse)
- Fever
- Abdominal pain

Syphilis

Transmission is sexual via secretions, kissing, or skin abrasions, or from mom to infant in utero.

- 1°—chancre @ site of exposure; incubates 1 wk to 3 months; highly contagious; buttonlike papule (painless)
- 2°—rash (palms & soles), constitutional symptoms; nausea, loss of appetite, fever, sore throat, stomatitis, inflamed eyes, red-brown 2–3 cm lesions on genitals (foul, contagious discharge)
- 3°—destructive lesions to CV & neural systems

HIV (Human Immunodeficiency Virus)
AIDS (Acquired Immunodeficiency Syndrome)

Transmission: blood products, CSF, semen, vaginal secretions, mom to child

Early HIV Signs	Advanced HIV Signs
■ Fever, night sweats ■ Chronic diarrhea ■ Oral infections ■ Vaginal candidiasis ■ Cough ■ SOB ■ Skin/nail changes	■ Kaposi's sarcoma–multiple purple skin blotches ■ Persistent cough ■ Fever, night sweats ■ Easy bruising ■ Thrush ■ Muscle weakness ■ Comorbidities: TB, pneumonia, lymphoma, herpes, toxoplasmosis

Source: Goodman C & Snyder T (2000).

Neuropsychiatric Disorders

Signs & Symptoms of Depression

- Sadness; frequent/unexplained crying
- Feelings of guilt, helplessness, or hopelessness
- Suicide ideations
- Problems sleeping
- Fatigue or decreased energy; apathy
- Loss of appetite; weight loss/gain
- Difficulty concentrating, remembering, & making decisions
- Bipolar disorder (manic-depression)—Peak onset is late teens with equal males/females with a strong genetic component. It may be a neurotransmitter abnormality.

Eating Disorders

Note: Bradycardia in a thin adolescent is a red flag for anorexia

Anorexia	Bulimia
■ Under minimal body weight	■ Binge eating
■ Fear of being fat	■ Self-induced vomiting
■ Frequent starving	■ Laxatives, diuretics
■ Social withdrawal	■ Excessive exercise
■ Depressed	■ Overeating alternating
■ Insomnia	with period of starvation
■ ↑ Libido	■ Fear of fatness
■ Self-induced vomiting	■ May be obese
■ Excessive exercise	■ Erosion of dental enamel
■ Diuretics	■ Seizures
■ Amenorrhea	■ Weakness & fatigue
■ ↓ Cortisol, serotonin, growth	■ Lab–metabolic acidosis,
hormone, corticotropin-	↑ amylase, hypokalemia,
releasing factor	hypomagnesia
■ ↑ LH, FSH, TSH	
■ Bradycardia	
■ Hypotension	
■ Arrhythmias	
■ Dry skin, dental caries,	
anemia, osteoporosis	
■ Lab–hypokalemia, ↓ BUN,	
metabolic alkalosis	

Source: Boissonnault WG (2005).

Signs & Symptoms of Panic Disorder

■ Pounding tachycardia	■ Hand wringing
■ Chest pain	■ Perceptual distortions
■ Dizziness, nausea	■ Sense of terror
■ Difficulty breathing, SOB	■ Extreme fear of losing control
■ Bilateral numbness	■ Fear of dying
■ Tingling in face	■ Feeling of choking/smothering
■ Sweats or chills	■ Vertigo

HIV (Human Immunodeficiency Virus)
AIDS (Acquired Immunodeficiency Syndrome)

Transmission: blood products, CSF, semen, vaginal secretions, mom to child

Early HIV Signs	Advanced HIV Signs
■ Fever, night sweats ■ Chronic diarrhea ■ Oral infections ■ Vaginal candidiasis ■ Cough ■ SOB ■ Skin/nail changes	■ Kaposi's sarcoma–multiple purple skin blotches ■ Persistent cough ■ Fever, night sweats ■ Easy bruising ■ Thrush ■ Muscle weakness ■ Comorbidities: TB, pneumonia, lymphoma, herpes, toxoplasmosis

Source: Goodman C & Snyder T (2000).

Neuropsychiatric Disorders

Signs & Symptoms of Depression

- Sadness; frequent/unexplained crying
- Feelings of guilt, helplessness, or hopelessness
- Suicide ideations
- Problems sleeping
- Fatigue or decreased energy; apathy
- Loss of appetite; weight loss/gain
- Difficulty concentrating, remembering, & making decisions
- Bipolar disorder (manic-depression)—Peak onset is late teens with equal males/females with a strong genetic component. It may be a neurotransmitter abnormality.

Eating Disorders	
Note: Bradycardia in a thin adolescent is a red flag for anorexia	
Anorexia	**Bulimia**
■ Under minimal body weight ■ Fear of being fat ■ Frequent starving ■ Depressed ■ Social withdrawal ■ Insomnia ■ ↓ Libido ■ Self-induced vomiting ■ Excessive exercise ■ Diuretics ■ Amenorrhea ■ ↑ Cortisol, serotonin, growth hormone, corticotropin-releasing factor ■ ↓ LH, FSH, TSH ■ Bradycardia ■ Hypotension ■ Arrhythmias ■ Dry skin, dental caries, anemia, osteoporosis ■ Lab–hypokalemia, ↑ BUN, metabolic alkalosis	■ Binge eating ■ Self-induced vomiting ■ Laxatives, diuretics ■ Excessive exercise ■ Overeating alternating with period of starvation ■ Fear of fatness ■ May be obese ■ Erosion of dental enamel ■ Seizures ■ Weakness & fatigue ■ Lab–metabolic acidosis, ↓ amylase, hypokalemia, hypomagnesia

Source: Boissonnault WG (2005).

Signs & Symptoms of Panic Disorder

- ■ Pounding tachycardia
- ■ Chest pain
- ■ Dizziness, nausea
- ■ Difficulty breathing, SOB
- ■ Bilateral numbness
- ■ Tingling in face
- ■ Sweats or chills
- ■ Hand wringing
- ■ Perceptual distortions
- ■ Sense of terror
- ■ Extreme fear of losing control
- ■ Fear of dying
- ■ Feeling of choking/smothering
- ■ Vertigo

Obsessive-Compulsive Disorders

Medical brain disorder that causes problems in information processing. Typically manifests from preschool to age 40.

Types of Obsessions	Associated Compulsions
Contamination fears (germs, dirt, etc)	Washing
Imagining having harmed self/others	Repeating
Imagining losing control/aggressive urges	Checking
Intrusive sexual thoughts/urges	Touching
Excessive religious/moral doubt	Counting
Forbidden thoughts	Order/arranging
A need to have things "just so"	Hoarding/saving
A need to tell, ask, confess	Praying

Source: http://www.ocfoundation.org/

The Mood Disorder Questionnaire (MDQ)

Question:	Yes	No
1. Has there ever been a period of time when you were not your usual self and …		
■ you felt so good or so hyper that other people thought you were not your normal self or you were so hyper that you got into trouble?		
■ you were so irritable that you shouted at people or started fights or arguments?		
■ you felt much more self-confident than usual?		
■ you got much less sleep than usual and found that you didn't really miss it?		
■ you were more talkative or spoke much faster than usual?		
■ thoughts raced through your head or you couldn't slow your mind down?		
■ you were so easily distracted by things around you that you had trouble concentrating or staying on track?		
■ you had much more energy than usual?		
■ you were much more active or did many more things than usual?		
■ you were much more social or outgoing than usual, for example, you telephoned friends in the middle of the night?		
■ you were much more interested in sex than usual?		
■ you did things that were unusual for you or that other people might have thought were excessive, foolish, or risky?		
■ spending money got you or your family in trouble?		

(Continued text on following page)

The Mood Disorder Questionnaire (MDQ) (Continued)

Question:	Yes	No
2. If you checked YES to more than 1 of the above, have several of these ever happened during the same period of time?		
3. How much of a problem did any of these cause you –like being able to work; having family, money, or legal troubles; getting into arguments or fights?		
None Minor Moderate Severe problem		
4. Have any of your blood relatives (i.e., children, siblings, parents, grandparents, aunts, uncles) had manic-depressive illness or bipolar disorder?		
5. Has a health professional ever told you that you have manic-depressive illness or bipolar disorder?		

Scoring Algorithm:

All 3 of the following criteria **must** be met for a **Positive Screen**:

■■■ Question 1–7 of 13 "Yes" responses
■■ Question 2—"Yes" response
■ Question 3—"Moderate" or "Severe" response

Source: Hirschfeld RM et al (2000).

Other Pathology

Bacterial Meningitis = medical emergency (especially in children)

Infant	Adult
■ Fever	■ H/A, fever, chills
■ Lethargy (hypotonia)	■ Photophobia
■ Poor feeding	■ Vomiting, nausea
■ Vomiting	■ URI symptoms
■ Respiratory distress	■ Seizures in 20–30% of cases
■ Apnea	■ Confusion
■ Cyanosis	■ (+) Kernig sign = hip flexed to 90°, pain reproduced with knee extension
■ Paradoxic irritability (quiet when stationary & cries when held)	■ (+) Brudzinski sign = supine neck flexion reproduces pain
■ Seizures in 30–40% of cases	■ Stiff neck
	■ Sleepiness

Source: Boissonnault WG (2005).

Adolescent Cancer Screening

- Osteosarcoma
  - ■ Most common bone cancer in adolescence
  - ■ Occurs in boys $2 \times >$ girls
  - ■ Most common bones are femur, tibia, fibula
  - ■ Pain & swelling that gets worse with exercise or at night
  - ■ Pathology fx may eventually occur
- Leukemia
  - ■ Difficult to diagnose because of the similarity to normal childhood diseases
  - ■ Onset can be slow or rapid
  - ■ Fever & loss of appetite
  - ■ Pale skin & frequent bruising
  - ■ Enlarged cervical lymph nodes
  - ■ Abdominal protrusion, 2° enlargement of spleen & liver
  - ■ ↑ Irritability

- Pilocytic astrocytoma (peaks at 5–14 yo)
    - H/A–worse in AM
    - H/A ↑ with activity, Valsalva, stooping (↑ intracranial pressure)
    - Seizures
    - Visual changes
    - Vomiting
    - Ataxia
- Bone tumors (rare with good prognosis)
    - Located @ ends of long bones
    - Usually asymptomatic
    - Night pain unaffected by position
    - Swelling
    - Fever, night sweats
    - Fatigue, wt loss
- Hodgkin's disease–males > females (5:1)
    - Lymph nodes > 1 cm–tender, rubbery, firm (lasting longer than 4 wks)
    - Pruritis (greater @ night)
    - Fever, night sweats
    - Anorexia, anemia
    - Jaundice
    - Edema
    - Nonproductive cough, dyspnea
    - Chest pain
    - Cyanosis

Musculoskeletal Pathology

Ottawa Knee Rules

X-ray series of the *knee* is only required if the patient presents with any of the following criteria:

- > 55 years old
- Isolated tenderness of the patella
- Tenderness of the head of the fibula
- Inability to flex > 90 degrees
- Inability to bear weight (4 steps) *both* immediately after injury & in emergency department (regardless of limping)

Ottawa Ankle Rules

X-ray series of the *ankle* is only required if the patient presents with any of the following criteria:

- Bone tenderness at posterior edge of the distal 6 cm of the medial malleolus
- Bone tenderness at posterior edge of the distal 6 cm of the lateral malleolus
- Totally unable to bear weight *both* immediately after injury & (for 4 steps) in the emergency department

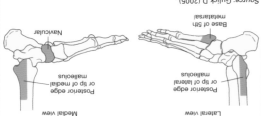

Lateral view
Posterior edge or tip of lateral malleolus
Base of fifth metatarsal

Medial view
Posterior edge or tip of medial malleolus
Navicular

Source: Gulick D (2005).

Ottawa Foot Rules

X-ray series of the *foot* is only required if the patient presents with any of the following criteria:

- Bone tenderness is at navicular
- Bone tenderness at the base of 5th MT
- Totally unable to bear weight *both* immediately after injury & (for 4 steps) in the emergency department

Osteoporosis

Substances that can ↓ bone density	**Risk factors ≥ 3 factors = ↑ risk**
■ Aluminum	■ Caucasian
■ Antiseizure meds	■ Female
■ Corticosteroids	■ > 65 years old
■ Cytotoxic meds	■ Substance abuse
■ ↑ Thyroxine	(smoking, alcohol)
■ Heparin	■ Lactose intolerance or
■ Caffeine	low Ca^{++} intake
■ Tobacco	■ Inactivity
	■ Thyroid, NSAIDs, steroids
	■ Family hx
	■ Kidney disease
	■ Thin stature/low body weight
	■ Early menopause

Signs & Symptoms
- Severe & localized T-L-spine pain
- ↑ Pain with prolonged posture
- ↑ Pain with Valsalva
- ↓ Pain in hook-lying
- Loss of ht > 1″
- Kyphosis
- Dowager's hump

Source: Boissonnault WG (2005).

Systemic Causes of Carpal Tunnel Syndrome

- DM
- Hormonal imbalance
- Pregnancy
- Gout
- Graves' disease (hyperthyroidism)
- Hyperparathyroidism
- Hypothyroidism
- Liver disease
- Oral contraceptives
- Obesity

Source: Goodman C & Snyder T (2000).

Fibromyalgia Syndrome

- Widespread pain for > 3 months
- Myalgia & AM stiffness
- Fatigue & sleep disturbance 2° ↓ GH released @ night
- Soft tissue swelling
- Headache, dyspnea, dizziness
- Hypersensitivity to light
- Dry eyes & mouth
- Presence of 11 of 18 tender points

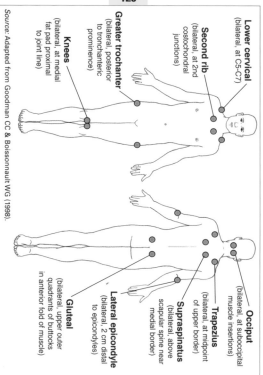

Lower cervical
(bilateral, at C5–C7)

Second rib
(bilateral, at 2nd
costochondral
junctions)

Greater trochanter
(bilateral, posterior
to trochanteric
prominence)

Knees
(bilateral, at medial
fat pad proximal
to joint line)

Occiput
(bilateral, at suboccipital
muscle insertions)

Trapezius
(bilateral, at midpoint
of upper border)

Supraspinatus
(bilateral, above
scapular spine near
medial border)

Lateral epicondyle
(bilateral, 2 cm distal
to epicondyles)

Gluteal
(bilateral, upper outer
quadrants of buttocks
in anterior fold of muscle)

Arthritic Changes		
OA	**RA**	**Gout**
■ Asymmetrical involvement	■ Symmetrical jt swelling	■ Affects only a few joints
■ Large wt-bearing joints	■ Small jts–hands, feet, wrist	■ Most common: 1st MTP, knee, wrist
■ Loss of jt surface integrity	■ Erythema & fever	■ Abrupt onset of severe pain
■ Formation of osteophytes	■ Intense pain after rest	■ Uric acid crystals in synovial fluid
■ Intra-articular loose bodies	■ Wt loss, nutritional deficiencies	■ ↑ Frequency with ↑ age
■ Soft tissue contractures	■ Loss of stamina & weakness	■ Males >females
■ ↓ ROM	■ ↑ Proteolytic enzymes	■ Usually begins @ night
■ Stiffness after activity	■ Enlarged spleen	
■ Deep ache	■ Lymphadenopathy	
	■ Heart & lung pathology	
	■ Jt subluxations	
	■ Vasculitis	
	■ Rheumatoid nodules	

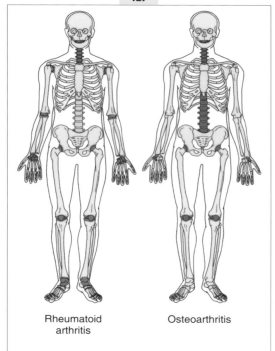

Rheumatoid arthritis

Osteoarthritis

Neuromuscular Pathology

Adverse Effects of Statins

- Loss of muscular coordination
- Trouble talking & enunciating words
- Loss of balance
- Loss of fine motor skills (difficulty writing)
- Trouble swallowing
- Constant fatigue
- Joint & muscle aches & stiffness
- Vertigo & disorientation
- Blinding headaches

Hypothesis: statins inhibit cholesterol production to ↑ LDLs & may be indirectly causing membrane degeneration

Possible Signs & Symptoms of a Brain Tumor

- H/A–↑ intracranial pressure
- Vomiting
- Visual changes
- Mentation changes
- Seizures
- Muscle weakness
- Bladder dysfunction
- Coordination changes
- (+) Babinski
- Clonus (ankle or wrist)

SCI Autonomic Dysreflexia

Exaggerated sympathetic reflex response in SCI patients

- Severe hypertension
- Bradycardia
- Headache
- Vasospasm, skin pallor & gooseflesh below the level of injury
- Arterial vasodilation, flushed skin, & profuse sweating above the level of injury

Cauda Equina Syndrome (CES)

This is a rare disorder (< 4 in 10,000) affecting the bundle of nerve roots (cauda equina) at the lower (lumbar) end of the spinal cord & is a surgical emergency. An extension of the brain, the nerve roots send/receive messages to/from the pelvic organs & lower limbs. CES occurs when the nerve roots are compressed & paralyzed, cutting off sensation & mov't. Nerve roots that control the function of the bladder & bowel are especially vulnerable to damage.

Signs & Symptoms

- B & B changes (poor sphincter tone)
- Saddle anesthesia (toilet paper feels different when wiping)
- Global or progressive LE weakness: $1°$ = toe ext & dorsi/plantarflexion
- Sensory deficits in feet (bilateral)
- ↓ Reflexes
- Pain radiating into both legs
- (−) Babinski sign
- (+) SLR

Myasthenia Gravis

Myasthenia Gravis comes from the Greek & Latin words meaning "grave muscular weakness." It is an immune problem with acetylcholine receptors blocked.
Primary onset: 20–30 yo ♀ > ♂ & > 50 yo ♂ > ♀

Signs & Symptoms

- Diplopia & ptosis = most common symptoms
- Proximal muscle weakness
- Problem controlling eye mov't & facial expressions
- Difficulty swallowing & chewing
- Dysarthria/dysphagia
- Change in voice quality
- No sensory changes or change in DTRs

The edrophonium chloride (Tensilon) test is performed by injecting this chemical into a vein. Improvement of strength immediately after the injection provides strong support for the diagnosis of MG.

Guillain Barré Syndrome (GBS)

Progressive demyelination of peripheral nerves resulting from an autoimmune response. Often occurs after viral or URI. Onset: Effects all ages but peaks 15-35 & 50-75 yo
♂ > ♀ 1.5:1

Signs & Symptoms

- Weakness—symmetrical LE > UE > respiratory
- Paresthesia start in toes & progress proximal (no loss of sensation)
- Pain = LB & buttocks
- Cranial nerves effected in 45-75% of cases
- Asymmetrical facial weakness, dysphasia, dysarthrias
- Unstable vital signs
- ↑ Reflexes & hypotonia
- Fever, nausea, fatigue

Amyotrophic Lateral Sclerosis (ALS)

A progressive, fatal, motor neuron disease, known as Lou Gehrig's disease, is hereditary (~5 per 100,000). Mean survival time with ALS is 3-5 years. Entire sensory system & intellect remain intact.

Signs & Symptoms	Conditions to Rule Out
■ Muscle weakness: hands, arms, legs	■ Lymphoma
■ Progressive weakness of muscles of speech, swallowing, & eventually breathing	■ Lyme disease
	■ Spinal cord compression
■ EMG—fibrillations & fasciculations	■ Heavy metal poisoning
■ Denervation atrophy	
■ Elevated muscle enzymes	
■ Painful UE cramps	

Multiple Sclerosis

Onset: 13–35 yo; women > men by 2:1
Disease of temperate climates—highest incidence = born in latitudes of 40–45°. Possible genetic risk.
Most common location of early lesions are sensory (numbness), pyramidal (LE weakness), cerebellar (double vision, vertigo), & visual pathways (blurred vision, loss of vision in one eye). Sclerotic plaques disseminate through the brain & spinal cord. Presentation is highly variable. The number of exacerbations per year is directly related to the progression of the disease. The younger the onset, the better the prognosis.

Signs & Symptoms

- Intermittent unilateral visual impairment
  - Blurring
  - Diplopia
- Paresthesias
- Ataxia
- Vertigo
- Fatigue
- Extremity weakness
- B & B changes
- Reports a sensation of compression around a limb
- Hyper-reflexia
- (+) Babinski
- Dysmetria
- Lhermitte's sign = electric sensation down the back with neck flexion
- Sensitivity to temperature changes
- LBP 2° trunk hypotonia

MS Classification

Type	Manifestation
Relapsing Remitting	Episode followed by recovery
Secondary Progressive	Steadily progressive pattern
Primary Progressive	Steady decline from onset
Progressive Relapsing	Progressive disease with exacerbation

Systemic Lupus Erythematosus

An autoimmune disease of unknown etiology that results in inflammation & damage to various organs.
Onset: 15–45 yo ♀ > ♂ 10–15:1
African (3× more common), Native-American, Asian > Caucasian

Signs & Symptoms

- Unexplained fever
- Swollen glands
- Constitutional symptoms
- Arthralgia—symmetrical
- Swollen joints
- Skin rash—"butterfly" pattern (cheeks)
- Chest pain upon deep breathing
- Extreme fatigue
- Photosensitivity
- Unusual hair loss
- Pale or purple fingers or toes from cold or stress (Raynaud's phenomenon)
- CNS px—seizures, h/a, peripheral neuropathy, CVA, OBS
- Mouth, nose, vaginal ulcers
- Symptoms get worse during menstruation

Complications of Lupus

- Seizures/psychosis
- Pleuritis/pericarditis
- Endocarditis/myocarditis
- Anemia
- Glomerulonephritis

Note: A severe side effect of the acne medication minocycline, is lupuslike symptoms.

Cardiovascular & Pulmonary Pathology

Clinical Signs of Pneumonia

- Fever, chills
- Chest pain
- SOB
- Cough
- Rust-colored sputum

Asthma

Triggers

- Respiratory infections
- Cigarette smoke/pollutants
- Allergic reactions
- Exercise
- Cold environments
- Stress

Signs & Symptoms

- Wheezing
- Prolonged expiration
- Difficulty breathing
- Cough
- SOB

Asthma Inhalers

- **Short-acting bronchodilator** = immediate symptom relief; e.g., albuterol (Proventil, Ventolin), pirbuterol (Maxair)
- **Long-acting bronchodilators** = up to 12 hrs of symptom relief; e.g., salmeterol (Serevent); formoterol (Foradil)
- **Corticosteroids** = long-term prevention of symptoms, may take up to 7 days for peak effectiveness; e.g., beclomethasone diproprionate (QVAR); fluticasone (Flovent); budesonide (Pulmicort); triamcinolone acetonide (Azmacort); flunisolide (AeroBid)
- **Nonsteroidals** = long-term prevention of inflammation; e.g., Cromolyn, nedocromil
- **Corticosteroid 1 bronchodilator** = long-acting combination; e.g., Advair

Anemia

Causes

- Chemotherapy
- GI bleed
- RA
- Lupus
- AIDS
- CA
- Surgery

Signs & Symptoms

- ↓ Hemoglobin
- ↓ Hematocrit
- Change in fingernail beds
- Pale skin color
- Fatigue
- ↓ DBP

Source: Goodman C & Snyder T (2000).

Transient Ischemic Attack (TIA)

Symptoms depend on cerebral vessel involved
- Anterior Cerebral Artery = LE > UE; frontal signs
- Middle Cerebral Artery = forearm, hand, & mouth affected
- Posterior Cerebral Artery = visual disturbances, graying out, blurring, fogging

Warning Signs of a Stroke
- Sudden weakness or numbness in face or extremities
- Loss of vision in 1 eye or dimness
- Difficulty with speech or understanding
- Sudden severe h/a
- Unexplained dizziness, unsteadiness or falls

Risk(s) for Hemorrhagic Stroke
- < 65 yo
- HTN
- Anomaly of a vessel
- Anticoagulation therapy
- Liver disease
- Recreational drug use
- Alcohol abuse

Pericarditis
- May be preceded by infection
- Fever
- Pain in supine, with inspiration/cough
- ↑ Pain with leaning forward
- ↓ HR & RR
- Neck vein distention

Clinical Signs of Hypertension
- Spontaneous epistaxis
- Occipital h/a
- Dizziness
- Visual changes
- Nocturnal urinary frequency
- Flushed face

Source: Goodman C & Snyder T (2000).

Signs & Symptoms of Congestive Heart Failure (CHF)

- SOB, dyspnea
- Sleeps sitting up
  2° orthopnea
- Enlarged liver
- LE edema

- Pleural effusion
- Scrotal edema
- Distended neck veins
- Tachycardia
- ↓ Renal perfusion

Onset & Duration of Various Forms of Nitroglycerin

Onset	Form	Duration
20–45 min	Oral	4–6 hrs
2–3 min	Buccal	3–5 hrs
1–3 min	Sublingual	30–60 min
30 min	Ointment	4–8 hrs
< 30 min	Patches	8–24 hrs

Source: Ciccone CD (2002).

Signs & Symptoms of MI in Men

- Substernal pressure, tightness, squeezing
- Pain unrelieved by position or nitroglycerin
- Dyspnea
- Nausea, vomiting, dizziness
- Palpitations, diaphoresis

Signs & Symptoms of MI in Women
(in order of frequency of occurrence)

Prodromal Symptoms Average = 5.71 ± 4.36	Acute Symptoms Average = 7.3 ± 4.8
■ Unusual fatigue (71%)	■ SOB (58%)
■ Sleep disturbance (48%)	■ Weakness (55%)
■ SOB (42%)	■ Unusual fatigue (43%)
■ Indigestion (39%)	■ Dizziness (39%)
■ Anxious (36%)	■ Cold sweat (39%)
■ Heart racing (27%)	■ Nausea (36%)
■ Weak/heavy arms (25%)	■ Weak/heavy arms (35%)
■ Changes in thinking or remembering (24%)	■ Arm aching (32%)
■ Vision changes (23%)	■ Hot or flushed (32%)
■ Loss of appetite (22%)	■ Indigestion (31%)
■ Hands/arms tingling (22%)	■ Centered high chest pain (31%)
■ Difficulty breathing @ PM (19%)	■ Racing heart (23%)
■ Arm aching (19%)	■ Left arm/shoulder pain (22%)
■ Cough (18%)	■ Scapula pain (21%)
■ ↑ Frequency of h/a (13%)	■ Arm/hand tingling (21%)
■ Centered high chest pain (14%)	■ General chest pain (20%)
■ Scapula pain (13%)	■ Loss of appetite (19%)
■ General chest pain (13%)	■ Vomiting (19%)
■ Left shoulder/arm pain (12%)	■ Neck/throat pain (16%)
■ Numbness both hands (11%)	■ H/A (15%)
■ Left breast pain (9%)	■ Left breast pain (15%)
■ ↑ Intensity of h/a (9%)	■ Vision change (13%)
	■ Bilateral arm pain (12%)
	■ Cough (11%)
	■ Top of shoulder pain (10%)
	■ Jaw/teeth pain (10%)

Source: McSweeney JC, et al. (2003).

Note: Current literature has revealed that the signs & symptoms of MI may be significantly different for men & women. Thus, the differentiation of these characteristics are presented by gender.

Wells Clinical Score for Deep Vein Thrombosis

Clinical Parameter Score	Score
Active cancer (treatment ongoing or within 6 months)	+ 1
Paralysis or recent immobilization of LE	+ 1
Recently bedridden for > 3 days or major surgery < 4 weeks	+ 1
Localized tenderness along the distribution of the deep venous system	+ 1
Entire leg swelling	+ 1
Calf swelling > 3 cm compared to the asymptomatic leg	+ 1
Pitting edema (> asymptomatic leg)	+ 1
Previous DVT documented	+ 1
Collateral superficial veins (nonvaricose)	+ 1
Alternative diagnosis (as likely or > that of DVT)	− 2
Total Score	
High probability	≥ 3
Moderate probability	1–2
Low probability	≤ 0

Source: Anand SS, Wells PS, Hunt D, et al. (1998).

Additional Risks of DVT

- AIDS
- Varicose veins
- Pacemakers
- Pregnancy
- Obesity
- Acute myocardial infarction
- Long airline flights
- Recent central venous catheterization
- Blood type A
- Antithrombin deficiency
- Oral contraceptives

Sources of Emboli

Arterial	Venous
■ Carotid artery 2° atherosclerosis	■ Venous catheterization
■ Left atrium 2° atrial fibrillation	■ Pulmonary system 2° infarct
■ Mitral valve	■ Injections, i.e., air
■ Aortic valve	■ Amniotic fluid
■ Left ventricle 2° MI	■ Renal system 2° CA
■ Aorta 2° atherosclerosis	■ Fat emboli 2° fx
■ Aorta 2° aneurysm	■ LE thrombosis 2° immobilization
■ Iliac artery 2° aneurysm or atherosclerosis	

Signs & Symptoms of a Pulmonary Embolus

- ■ Anginalike pain or crushing chest pain
- ■ Dyspnea, wheezing, rales
- ■ Hemoptysis, chronic cough
- ■ ↑ BP
- ■ Fever
- ■ Tachypnea (> 16/min)
- ■ Tachycardia (> 100/min)
- ■ Diaphoresis

Source: Rubin E & Faber JL (1994).

Signs & Symptoms of Pathology of the Spleen

- ■ Hx of anemia
- ■ Gingivitis, sore/bleeding gums
- ■ Painful tongue
- ■ Fatigue
- ■ Vertigo/tinnitus
- ■ Low resistance to colds/infections
- ■ Muscle tension h/a
- ■ Tachycardia
- ■ Pale skin

Integumentary Pathology

Herpes Zoster (shingles)

- 2/3 of patients are > 50 yo
- Pain, tenderness, & paraesthesia in the dermatome may be present 3–5 days before vesicular eruption
- Prodromal pain may mimic cardiac or pleural pain
- Erythema & vesicles follow a dermatomal distribution
- Pustular vesicles from crusts lasting 2–3 weeks
- Thoracic (50%) & ophthalmic division of trigeminal nerve are most commonly affected regions
- Contagious via respiratory droplets or direct contact with blisters

Cellulitis

A serious bacterial infection of the skin that can spread to lymph nodes & bloodstream. Cellulitis is not contagious.

People at Risk

- DM
- Circulatory px
- Liver disease
- Eczema
- Psoriasis
- Chickenpox
- Severe acne
- Hx of CHF

Signs & Symptoms

- Pain, swelling, warmth
- Erythema with streaks & vague borders
- Fever & chills
- Recent skin disruption
- Headache
- Low BP
- Enlarged lymph nodes
- Small red spots appear on top of reddened skin

Eczema/Dermatitis

A noninfective inflammatory skin condition. Eczema is Greek for "boil over" & this describes the blistering pattern of the skin.

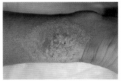

Source: From Barankin B & Freiman A (2006).

Occupational Hazards for Dermatitis

Bakers	Flour, flavorings, sugar, enzymes, detergent
Builders	Cement, rubber, glass wool, rubber, resin, acids, wood
Cleaners	Detergents, solvents, rubber gloves, fragrances
Electronics	Solder, solvents, fiberglass, acrylate, resins
Farmers/vets	Disinfectant, rubber, antibiotics, plants, preservatives, animal secretions
Food service	Specific foods, rubber gloves, spices, preservatives, detergent
Hair stylist	Shampoo, bleach, perm lotions, dyes, fragrances
Metal workers	Oils, cleanser, solvents, preservatives, Ni, Cr, Co
Office workers	Paper, fiberglass, rubber, dyes, glues, Ni
Textile workers	Solvents, formaldehyde, dyes, bleach, Ni

Source: Gawkrodger DJ (2003).

Psoriasis

- Variable severity
- Peak onset = 2nd, 3rd, & 6th decades
- Chronic skin disease with red patches covered with white scales
- Rash usually occurs on the extensor surfaces (elbows & knees), scalp, nails
- Psoriatic arthritis may also develop
- Beta blockers, lithium, & antimalarial drugs can bring on or make psoriasis worse

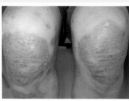

Source: From Barankin B & Freiman A (2006).

Skin Cancers

Risk factors: Significant hx of sun exposure & fair skin, light hair & eyes

Basal Cell

Warning signs:

- A sore that remains open for ≥ 3 wks
- A reddish patch (may crust or itch)
- A shiny bump or nodule
- A pink growth with an elevated rolled border & a crusted indentation
- A scarlike area that is white & waxy

Prognosis:

- Painless & slow-growing
- Rx = radiation &/or excision
- Seldom metastasizes

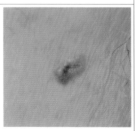

Source: From Barankin B & Freiman A (2006).

Squamous Cell

Warning signs:

- Wartlike growth that crusts & bleeds
- Scaly red patch with irregular borders
- A open sore that persists for weeks

Prognosis:

- Good if surgical excision & topical agents remove cells before infiltration to underlying tissue & metastasis into lymph channels

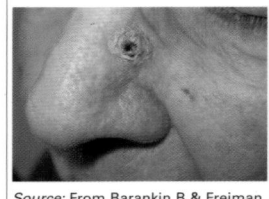

Source: From Barankin B & Freiman A (2006).

Malignant melanoma

Warning signs (ABCDE):

- Asymmetrical shape of a mole
- Border is irregular with jagged edges
- Color is varied/mixed
- Diameter is ≥ 7 mm
- Evolving
- Itching, crusting, bleeding may occur

Prognosis:

- Strongly influenced by the stage of the melanoma– range is local surgery to chemotherapy/radiation

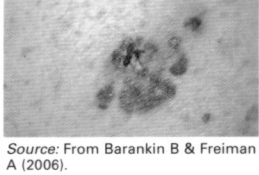

Source: From Barankin B & Freiman A (2006).

Source: http://www.skincancer.org.

Lyme Disease

Note: This is a multisystemic inflammatory condition. The transmission of the tick spirochete takes ~24 hrs. Blood work is used to confirm the disease, not to diagnose it. Transplacental transmission has been documented. Clinician should r/o GBS, MS, & FMS.

Early Localized Stage

■ Rash & onset of erythema in 7–14 days (range = 3–30 days)
■ Rash may be solid red expanding rash or a central spot with rings (bull's-eye)
■ Average diameter of rash is 5–6"
■ Rash may or may not be warm to palpation
■ Rash is usually not painful or itchy
■ Fever
■ Malaise
■ Headache
■ Muscle aches; joint pain

Early Disseminated Stage

■ ≥ 2 rashes not @ the bite site
■ Migrating pain
■ Headache; stiff neck; facial palsy
■ Numbness/tingling into extremities
■ Abnormal pulse
■ Sore throat
■ Visual changes
■ 100–102° fever
■ Severe fatigue

Late Stage

■ Arthritis of 1–2 larger joints
■ Neurological changes—disorientation, confusion, dizziness, mental "fog," numbness in extremities
■ Visual impairment
■ Cardiac irregularities

Source: American Lyme Disease Foundation.

Gastrointestinal Pathology

Strep Infection–Strep Throat

Self-limiting pathology lasting 3–5 days

- Sore throat
- Malaise
- Fever
- N/A

Staph Infection

Gram Negative	Gram Positive
Usually introduced via medical devices:	■ Boils, styes, carbuncles, osteomyelitis
■ IV	■ Infected burns
■ Heart valves	■ Infected surgical wounds
■ Pacemakers	■ Respiratory tract infections
■ Prostheses	■ Bacterial arthritis
■ Shunts	■ Septicemia
■ Catheters	■ Bacterial endocarditis
	■ Toxic shock
	■ Food poisoning

Ulcers

- Hx of NSAID use or presence of *H. pylori* infection
- Dull gnawing/burning into midline T6–12 & radiating suprascapula
- Antacids provide temporary relief
- Nausea, coffee-grounds vomitus
- Bloody or black-tarry stools (melena)
- May have weeks of remission

Gastric	Duodenal
30–60 min after a meal	2–3 hrs after a meal
Epigastric cramping	
Localized tenderness	
① UQ	⑭ of midline

Hernia

Risk Factors

- Surgery
- Heavy lifting
- Absence of linea alba
- Pregnancy

Signs & Symptoms

- Visible bulge
- Burning or dull ache
- Anterior hip pain (inguinal/femoral sheath hernia)
- Nausea, vomiting
- ↑ Pain with Valsalva, cough
- (+) Hip scour test due to compression of hernia

Gallbladder Pathology

Primary Risk Factors (6 Fs)

- Female
- Fair
- Flatulent
- Forty
- Fat
- Fertile

Signs & Symptoms

- Ⓡ UQ, scapula pain
- Symptoms ↑ after a fatty meal
- Pain does not respond to analgesics
- Abdominal bloating
- Excessive belching
- Clay-colored stools
- Vomiting, nausea
- Jaundice (small %)
- (+) Murphy's sign = inspiration inhibited by pain with palpation of Ⓡ UQ

Appendicitis

Onset: Most common in adolescents and young adults

Signs & Symptoms—in order of significant likelihood ratios	Differential Diagnosis
■ ® LQ pain, (+) McBurney's point => ® thigh/testicle ■ Nausea, vomiting, night sweats ■ Guarding of rectus abdominis ■ (+) Psoas sign ■ (+) Obturator sign ■ Low-grade fever ■ (+) Rebound tenderness ■ Position of relief: tense abdomen with FB or lie down with both knees to chest	■ ↓ Hemoglobin ■ ↓ Hematocrit ■ Change in fingernail beds ■ Pale skin color ■ Fatigue ■ ↓DBP

Source: American Family Physician
http://www.afp.org/afp/991101ap/2027.html

Bowel Pathology

Inflammatory Bowel (Crohn's or Ulcerative Colitis)	Irritable Bowel	Colon/Rectal Cancer
■ Joint arthralgia ■ Skin lesions (ankles, shins) ■ Light sensitivity ■ ↓ Pain with gas/BM ■ Anemia due to blood loss ■ Wt loss ■ Clubbing of fingers ■ Fever ■ Rectal bleeding ■ (+) Psoas test	■ Effects females in early adulthood ■ Stress related ■ Variable/ intermittent S&S ■ Abdominal cramps ■ Nausea & vomiting ■ Flatulence ■ Change in bowel patterns ■ Foul breath	■ Hemorrhoids ■ Rectal bleeding ■ Back pain referred to LEs ■ Change in bowel patterns ■ Nausea & vomiting ■ Wt loss ■ Fatigue & dyspnea due to iron deficiency ■ Red/mahogany stools

Hepatic Pathology

Hepatitis

Generalized Signs & Symptoms

- Nausea
- Vomiting
- Low-grade fever/chills
- Loss of appetite
- Lethargy
- Jaundice–skin & eyes
- Liver pain
- Dark urine
- Light-colored stools

Type	Incubation	Transmission	Cause
A	15–45 days	Fecal-oral (does not develop into chronic hepatitis)	Contaminated milk, water, shellfish, unsanitary conditions
B	2–3 months	Blood or body fluids Infants = carriers (can become chronic)	Contaminated needles, transfusion
C	15–90 days	Blood or body fluids (can become chronic)	Transfusion
D	25–75 days	Blood or body fluids	Occurs in presence of Hep B, IV drug use
E	20–80 days	Fecal-oral	Contaminated milk, water, shellfish
G	Unknown	Blood or body fluids	Transfusion, IV drug use

Endocrine Pathology

Breast Cancer

Risk Factors

- \> 40 years old
- Family hx
- Nonpregnancy
- Other cancers
- Fibrocystic disease

Signs & Symptoms

- Palpable mass
- Retraction of the nipple
- Dimpling of skin over mass
- Skin may be red, warm, edematous, firm, & painful over the mass
- Discharge from the nipple
- Pain with mov't of breast
- Fixation of mass to skin or chest wall
- Enlarged axillary lymph nodes

Signs & Symptoms of Diabetes

- ↓ Urination
- ↑ Thirst
- ↑ Hunger
- Fatigue, lethargy
- Wt loss
- Paresthesia (feet & hands)

Abnormal Blood Glucose

Hypoglycemia	Hyperglycemia
Blood glucose < 50-60 mg/dL	Blood glucose > 180 mg/dL
Skin is pale, cool, diaphoretic	Skin is dry & flushed
Disoriented or agitated	Fruity breath odor
Headache	Blurred vision
Blurred vision	Dizziness
Slurred speech	Weakness
Tachycardic with palpitations	Nausea
Weak/shaky	Vomiting
Lip/tongue numbness	Cramping
LOC	Increased urination
	LOC/seizure

Pancreatitis

Signs & Symptoms
- Severe epigastric & abdominal pain (most common = Ⓛ UQ)
- Pain radiates to the back
- Pain ↑ in supine & ↓ in sitting or leaning forward
- Abdominal distention, constipation, flatulence
- Tachycardic, hypotensive
- Nausea & vomiting
- Cool, clammy skin & fever
- Mild jaundice after 24 hours
- Pain after a large meal or ETOH consumption

Cushing Syndrome

Adrenal gland dysfunction

- Emotional disturbance
- Moon face
- Osteoporosis
- HTN
- Amenorrhea
- Muscle weakness
- Buffalo hump
- ↑ Facial hair
- Obesity
- Thin/wrinkled skin
- Purpura
- Skin ulcers/poor healing

Parathyroidism

Hypoparathyroidism	Hyperparathyroidism
■ Hypocalcemia ■ Irritability ■ Cardiac arrhythmia ■ Skeletal muscle twitching ■ Dry, scaly skin ■ Pigment changes ■ Thin hair ■ Brittle nails ■ (+) Chvostek's sign = twitching of facial mm with tapping of facial nerve in front of ear	■ ↑ DTRs ■ Fatigue, drowsiness ■ Proximal weakness ■ Arthralgia/myalgia ■ GI px/peptic ulcer ■ Kidney stones ■ Pancreatitis ■ Gout ■ Mental slowing or memory px ■ Emotional disorders ■ Hypercalcemia

Hyperthyroidism (Graves' Disease)

Signs in Order of Frequency of Occurrence:

Patients ≥ 70 years of age	Patients ≤ 50 years of age
■ Tachycardia	■ Tachycardia
■ Fatigue	■ Hyperactive reflexes
■ Weight loss	■ ↓ Sweating
■ Tremor	■ Heat intolerance
■ Dyspnea	■ Fatigue
■ Apathy	■ Tremor
■ Anorexia	■ Nervousness
■ Nervousness	■ Anorexia
■ Hyperactive reflexes	■ Weakness
■ Weakness	■ ↓ Appetite
■ Depression	■ Polydipsia
■ ↓ Sweating	■ Weight loss
■ Polydipsia	■ Dyspnea
■ Diarrhea	■ Diarrhea
■ Confusion	■ Apathy
■ Muscular atrophy	■ Depression
■ Heat intolerance	■ Muscular atrophy
■ Constipation	■ Anorexia

Source: Trivalle C, et al. (1996).

Hypothyroidism

■ ↑ Basal metabolic rate	■ Muscle/joint pain
■ Cold intolerance	■ Proximal weakness
■ Dry skin	■ Lethargy, depression, apathy
■ Brittle nails	■ Confusion
■ Sparse/coarse hair	■ Weight gain
■ Peripheral edema	■ Edema around the eyes
■ Jt effusion with Ca++ deposits	■ Loss of lateral eyebrow
■ Carpal tunnel syndrome	■ Cardiomegaly
■ Slow healing	■ Constipation
■ Hoarseness	
■ PR < 60 in untrained person	

Gout

- Rapid onset of sudden severe pain
- Inflammation of 1st MTP, knee, wrist, or elbow
- Redness, swelling
- Tenderness, hypersensitivity
- Fever, chills
- Yellowish-white papules on the fingertips, ears, elbows, & knuckles
- **Note:** Some diuretics used to treat CHF can cause gout.

Acromegaly

40–45 yrs old; insidious onset of excessive GH; most cases are due to pituitary adenoma

Signs & Symptoms

- Enlargement of hands & feet
- Barrel chested
- Broad/bulbous nose
- Protruding lower jaw
- Slanting forehead
- Teeth become splayed making chewing difficult
- Enlarged larynx that deepens voice
- Vertebral changes resulting in kyphosis & DJD
- Enlargement of all organs
- Development of DM (2° abnormal glucose tolerance)
- H/A & HTN
- Optic & CN palsies
- Excessive sweating (2° hypertrophic sebaceous glands)
- Wt gain
- Thickened skin
- Goiter
- Sexual dysfunction in males

Urogenital Pathology

5 Major Signs & Symptoms of Urinary Tract Pathology

1. Blood in urine (hematuria)
2. Edema–fluid retention
3. Pain–percussion over kidneys
4. Enlargement of kidneys
5. Anemia

Cystitis-Pyelonephritis (UTI)

- Pain with micturition
- Leukocytes & bacteria in urine (white casts)
- Cloudy urine
- Back pain
- Fever, chills
- Nausea
- Loss of appetite
- Pain with percussion over kidneys

Factors that Contribute to Urinary Incontinence

- UTIs
- Vaginal infection
- Constipation
- Enlarged prostate
- Damage to nerves of the bladder, e.g., Parkinson's
- Weak bladder muscles
- Overactive bladder muscles
- Medications
- Childbirth
- Surgery or trauma
- Normal pressure hydrocephalus

Types of Urinary Incontinence

- **Stress incontinence**: occurs when urine leaks during exercise, coughing, sneezing, laughing, lifting; most common in young or middle-aged women when pelvic muscle are weakened by childbirth or surgery
- **Urge incontinence**: urge comes on quickly & unable to get to the toilet in time; common in people who have had a CVA, DM, or Alzheimer's, Parkinson's, MS
- **Overflow incontinence**: constant urine dripping due to an overfull bladder; common in SCI, DM, & prostate px
- **Functional incontinence**: occurs in the disabled or aging patient when mobility limits the ability to get to the toilet in time

Kidney Stones

Risk Factors

- Males 4× > Females
- Caucasians 3× > Blacks
- 20–40 yrs old
- High-protein, low-fiber diet
- Dehydration
- Poor mobility
- Family hx

Signs & Symptoms

- Pain @ costovertebral angle
- Intermittent, excruciating pain into ipsilateral genitals
- Ureter spasms radiate into medial thigh
- Chills, nausea, vomiting
- Frequent urge to urinate
- Burning sensation with urination
- Bloody, cloudy, smelly urine

Source: http://hcdz.bupa.co.uk/fact.sheets/html/kidney_stones.html.

Endometriosis

Part of the spectrum of Pelvic Inflammatory Disease (PID)

- 30–40 yo
- Worse premenstrually & during menses
- Pain with intercourse
- Recurrent lumbosacral pain
- Infertility

Ectopic Pregnancy

Risk Factors

- History of pelvic inflammatory disease
- Endometriosis
- History of pelvic surgery
- Previous history of ectopic pregnancy

Signs & Symptoms

- Lower abdominal pain
- Pelvic or LB pain
- Pain referring into the shoulder girdle
- Rebound tenderness

Note: Fallopian tube typically ruptures by 12th week of pregnancy.

Sexually Transmitted Diseases (STD)

Genital Herpes
- Tingling, itching, genital pain
- Eruption of small pustules & vesicles
- Lesion rupture @ ~ 5 day to wet ulcers
- Dysuria & urine retention
- Fever, h/a, malaise, muscle ache, lymphadenopathy

Candidiasis = yeast infection, thrush
- Results from antibiotic therapy, ↑ hormone levels (pregnancy, oral contraceptives), DM

Gonorrhea
Transmitted via sexual intercourse or from mom to infant at birth (3–5 day incubation period)
- Urethral pain, dysuria
- Discharge
- Dyspareunia
- Vaginal bleeding (unusual or after intercourse)
- Fever
- Abdominal pain

Syphilis
Transmission is sexual via secretions, kissing, or skin abrasions or from mom to infant in utero
- 1°—chancre @ site of exposure; incubates 1 wk to 3 months; highly contagious; buttonlike papule (painless)
- 2°—rash (palms & soles), constitutional symptoms, nausea, loss of appetite, fever, sore throat, stomatitis, inflamed eyes, red-brown 2–3 cm lesions on genitals (foul, contagious discharge)
- 3°—destructive lesions to CV & neural systems

HIV (Human Immunodeficiency Virus)
AIDS (Acquired Immunodeficiency Syndrome)

Transmission: blood products, CSF, semen, vaginal secretions, mom to child

Early HIV Signs	Advanced HIV Signs
■ Fever, night sweats ■ Chronic diarrhea ■ Oral infections ■ Vaginal candidiasis ■ Cough ■ SOB ■ Skin/nail changes	■ Kaposi's sarcoma–multiple purple skin blotches ■ Persistent cough ■ Fever, night sweats ■ Easy bruising ■ Thrush ■ Muscle weakness ■ Co-morbidities: TB, pneumonia, lymphoma, herpes, toxoplasmosis

Source: Goodman C & Snyder T (2000).

Opportunistic Infections 2° AIDS

- ■ Meningitis
- ■ Toxoplasmosis
- ■ Herpes simplex
- ■ Candidiasis
- ■ Cytomegalovirus

- ■ *Staphylococcus*
- ■ Scabies
- ■ HPV
- ■ *Salmonella*

Source: Rubin E & Faber JL (1994).

Other Pathology

Signs of Autonomic Dysreflexia

- ■ Sweating above lesion
- ■ ↑ BP
- ■ Throbbing h/a
- ■ Goose bumps above the level of the lesion

- ■ Visual changes
- ■ Apprehension w/o apparent cause
- ■ Change in HR

- ■ **Emergency intervention** = identify trigger ASAP & sit up to ↓ BP

Bacterial Meningitis = medical emergency

Adult Signs & Symptoms

- H/A, fever, chills
- Photophobia
- Vomiting, nausea
- URI symptoms
- Seizures in 20–30% of cases
- Confusion
- (+) Kernig sign = hip flexed to 90°, pain reproduced with knee extension
- (+) Brudzinski sign = supine neck flexion reproduces pain
- Stiff neck
- Sleepiness

Source: Boissonnault WG (2005).

Non-Hodgkin's Lymphoma

- Peak incidence is 20–24 yrs of age
- Appearance of swollen glands in neck, axilla, groin
- Nonpainful & unresponsive to antibiotics
- Loss of appetite, nausea, vomiting, indigestion, wt loss
- Enlargement of liver, spleen, abdominal lymph nodes
- LBP referred to LE
- Anemia
- Night sweats & recurring fevers

Symptoms of Metastases by System

Pulmonary

- Cough
- Dyspnea
- Pleural pain
- Onset of wheezing

CNS

- Confusion, change in memory
- Blurred vision
- Depression
- Headache
- Irritability
- Balance px
- Drowsy
- Weakness

Skeletal (vertebrae, pelvis, ribs, femur)

- Significant pain relief with aspirin
- Pain @ night
- Prior hx of cancer
- Pain with weight-bearing

Signs & Symptoms Associated with the Most Common Primary Sites of Metastatic Tumors

Lung*	Prostate	Renal	Breast	Colon
> 60 yrs old	> 50 yrs old	55–60 yrs old	20–50 yrs old & > 65	>50 yrs old
Smoker	L/S pain	Hematuria	Nipple discharge	Abdominal pain
Shoulder, chest & C-spine pain	Frequent urination	Wt loss	Dimpling of breast	L/S pain
TOS symptoms	Weak urine stream	Malaise	Palpable mass	Change in bowel habits
Chronic cough	Difficulty starting urination	Fever		Bloody stools
Bloody sputum		Palpable posterior lateral abdominal mass		Wt loss
Malaise				Pain unaffected by position
Wt loss				
Fever				
Dyspnea				
Wheezing				

Note: Screening for metastasis to the spine can be done by attempting to provoke a sharp, localized pain with percussion with a reflex hammer over the spinous processes

*Pancoast tumor-mimics TOS, pain in ulnar distribution, intrinsic hand atrophy, UE venous distention

Source: Boissannault WG & Bass C (1990).

Physiological Changes with Pregnancy

Musculoskeletal

- ↑ BMR
- Weight gain of 20–25 lbs
- ↑ Rib cage circumference
- ↓ Spinal curves
- ↑ Ligamentous laxity
- Postural changes
- Change in center of gravity

Cardiovascular

- ↑ Blood volume
- ↑ RBC mass
- Iron deficiency
- ↑ Leukocyte count
- ↑ Coagulation factors
- ↑ Cardiac capacity
- ↑ Size of heart
- ↑ Cardiac output & ↑ HR

Pulmonary

- Voice changes
- Difficulty breathing through the nose
- ↑ Pulmonary dead space
- ↓ Residual volume
- ↑ Tidal volume
- ↑ Alveolar ventilation
- ↑ Respiratory rate
- ↑ O_2 consumption
- ↑ CO_2 output

Integumentary

- Vascular spiders
- Palmar erythema
- ↑ Sweating
- Striae gravidarum (stretch marks)
- Hyperpigmentation

Gastrointestinal

- ↓ pH of oral cavity with ↑ risk of tooth decay
- Tender/bleeding gums
- Gastric reflux
- ↓ GI motility
- ↑ Water absorption resulting in constipation
- ↓ Risk of gallstones

Endocrine

- Enlarged adrenal & thyroid glands
- Enlarged parathyroid & pituitary glands

Urogenital

- ↑ Urinary stasis with ↑ risk of infection
- ↑ Glomerular filtration rate
- Obstruction of uterus on inferior vena cava resulting in LE edema
- ↑ Urinary output

Source: Boissonnault WG (2005).

Precautions During Pregnancy

- Avoid x-ray exposure in 1st trimester
- Avoid supine for more than a few minutes after 4th month
- Avoid rapid, uncontrolled bouncing mov'ts
- Avoid overheating
- Avoid electrical stimulation & heating modalities to the abdominal region
- Avoid prone lying in the 3rd trimester
- Avoid taking aspirin, NSAIDs, & decongestants

Red Flags When Exercising During Pregnancy

- Calf swelling or pain
- Chest pain
- Leakage of amniotic fluid
- Premature labor
- ↓ Fetal mov't
- Dizziness/headache
- Vaginal bleeding

Musculoskeletal Complications

- LBP, SI px, nerve entrapment due to ↑ fluid volume (CTS)
- Mm cramps secondary to uterine pressure resulting in LE ischemia
- Pubic symphysis dysfunction
- Diastasis recti abdominis
- Restless leg syndrome (iron deficiency)

Cardiovascular & Pulmonary Complications

- Preeclampsia = rapidly progressive disorder that occurs after 20 weeks of pregnancy–h/a, blurred vision, edema, ↑ BP, proteinuria
- DVT
- Dyspnea
- Pregnancy-induced hypertension = h/a, blurred vision
- LE edema & varicose veins

Integumentary Complications

- Hyperpigmentation
- Palmar erythema
- Dermatoses

Gastrointestinal Complications

- GI px = nausea & vomiting may lead to dehydration, hypokalemia, & wt loss
- ↓ Motility may result in constipation
- Heartburn/gastric reflux
- Hemorrhoids
- ↑ Risk of gallstones
- *Toxoplasma gondii* (toxoplasmosis)–parasite–can be transmitted across the placenta

Hepatic Complications

- Although the liver is affected by physiological changes during pregnancy & the bilirubin excretion may be challenging in the 2nd half of pregnancy, liver tests are rarely abnormal.
- Liver pathology may be preexisting or nonpregnancy-related problems can develop, e.g., viral hepatitis or toxic hepatitis.

Hepatitis

Generalized Signs & Symptoms

- Nausea
- Vomiting
- Low-grade fever/chills
- Loss of appetite
- Lethargy
- Jaundice–skin & eyes
- Liver pain
- Dark urine
- Light-colored stools

Intrahepatic Cholestasis of Pregnancy
(Abnormalities in the flow of bile)

- Skin itching–most severe on palms of hands & soles of feet
- Jaundice–skin & whites of eyes

Endocrine Complications

Breast Cancer

Risk Factors

- >40 years old
- Family hx
- Nonpregnancy
- Other cancers
- Fibrocystic disease

Signs & Symptoms

- Palpable mass
- Enlarged axillary lymph nodes
- Retraction of the nipple
- Fixation of mass to skin or chest wall
- Dimpling of skin over mass
- Skin may be red, warm, edematous, firm, & painful over the mass
- Discharge from the nipple
- Pain with mov't of breast

Mastitis (inflammation of the breast)

Etiology

- Engorgement of breasts during nursing
- Plugged duct
- Infection

Signs & Symptoms

- Local breast tenderness & redness
- Edema
- Fever

Urogenital Complications

Ectopic Pregnancy

Risk Factors

- History of pelvic inflammatory disease
- Endometriosis
- History of pelvic surgery
- Previous history of ectopic pregnancy

Signs & Symptoms

- Lower abdominal pain
- Pelvic or LB pain
- Pain referring into the shoulder girdle
- Rebound tenderness

Note: Fallopian tube will typically rupture by the 12th week of pregnancy.

Placenta Abruption

Risk Factors

- Pregnant after age 35
- Has had > 4 children
- Pregnant with twins/triplets
- Has ↑ BP
- Use of cocaine

- Cigarette smoking
- Has diabetes
- Had a previous abruption
- Trauma

Signs & Symptoms

- Contractions that don't stop
- Pain in the uterus
- Abdominal or back pain

- ↓ Fetal mov'ts
- Blood in the amniotic fluid
- Vaginal bleeding

Source: http://folsomobgyn.com/placental_abruption.htm.

Cystitis-Pyelonephritis (UTI)

- Pain with micturition
- Leukocytes & bacteria in urine (white casts)
- Cloudy urine
- Back pain

- Fever, chills
- Nausea
- Loss of appetite
- Pain with percussion over kidneys

Sexually Transmitted Diseases (STDs)

Genital Herpes

- Tingling, itching, genital pain
- Eruption of small pustules & vesicles
- Lesion rupture @ ~ 5 day to wet ulcers
- Dysuria & urine retention
- Fever, h/a, malaise, muscle ache, lymphadenopathy

Candidiasis = yeast infection, thrush

- Results from antibiotic therapy, ↑ hormone levels (pregnancy, oral contraceptives), DM

Gonorrhea

Transmitted via sexual intercourse or from mom to infant at birth (3–5 day incubation period)

- Urethral pain, dysuria
- Discharge
- Dyspareunia
- Vaginal bleeding (unusual or after intercourse)
- Fever
- Abdominal pain

Syphilis

Transmission is sexual via secretions, kissing, or skin abrasions or from mom to infant in utero

- 1°–chancre @ site of exposure; incubates 1 wk to 3 months; highly contagious; buttonlike papule (painless)
- 2°–rash (palms & soles), constitutional symptoms, nausea, loss of appetite, fever, sore throat, stomatitis, inflamed eyes, red-brown 2–3 cm lesions on genitals (foul, contagious discharge)
- 3°–destructive lesions to CV & neural systems

Other Complications

- Cytomegalovirus (CMV)–member of the herpes family of viruses with mononucleosis-like symptoms; can be transmitted to the fetus & result in birth defects

Edinburgh Postnatal Depression Scale (EPDS)

Instructions: Check the response that comes closest to how you have been feeling in the past 7 days, not just how you feel today. Please complete all 10 items.

I have been able to laugh & see the funny side of things.
— As much as I always could
— Not quite so much now
— Definitely not so much now
— Not at all

I have looked forward with enjoyment to things.
— As much as I ever did
— Rather less than I used to
— Definitely less than I used to
— Hardly at all

I have blamed myself unnecessarily when things went wrong.
— No, never
— Not very often
— Yes, some of the time
— Yes, most of the time

I have been anxious or worried for no good reason.
— No, not at all
— Hardly ever
— Yes, sometimes
— Yes, very often

I have felt scared or panicky for no very good reason.
— No, not at all
— No, not much
— Yes, sometimes
— Yes, quite a lot

Things have been getting on top of me.
— No, I have been coping as well as ever
— No, most of the time I have coped quite well
— Yes, sometimes I haven't been coping as well as usual
— Yes, most of the time I haven't been able to cope at all

(Continued text on following page)

Edinburgh Postnatal Depression Scale (EPDS) *(Continued)*

I have been so unhappy that I have had difficulty sleeping.	I have felt sad or miserable.
– No, not at all	– No, not at all
– Not very often	– Not very often
– Yes, sometimes	– Yes, quite often
– Yes, most of the time	– Yes, most of the time

I have been so unhappy that I have been crying.	The thought of harming myself has occurred to me.
– No, never	– Never
– Only occasionally	– Hardly ever
– Yes, quite often	– Sometimes
– Yes, most of the time	– Yes, quite often

Score:

Scoring: The EPDS may be used at 6–8 weeks postpartum as a screening tool for Postpartum Depression (PPD). Categories are scored 0, 1, 2, and 3 according to increasing severity of symptoms. The total score is the sum of all 10 categories. Sensitivity = 86%; Specificity = 78%

- 0–8 points = low probability of depression
- 8–12 points = most likely just dealing with life with a new baby/baby blues
- 13–14 points = signs leading to the possibility of PPD; take preventative measures
- 15 + points = high probability of experiencing clinical PPD; take preventative measures

Source: Cox JL, Holden JM & Sagovsky R (1987).

Physiologic Changes with Aging

Musculoskeletal

- ↓ Muscle mass (↓ type II = FT) & strength
- ↓ Motor unit recruitment
- ↓ Speed of mov't
- ↓ Joint flexibility
- ↓ Bone mass & strength
- Cartilage degeneration

Neural

- ↓ Conduction = altered pain
- ↓ Enzymatic activity
- ↓ Reflexes
- ↑ Postural sway
- ↓ Responsiveness
- Change in sleep patterns

Cardiovascular

- ↓ Cardiac output
- ↑ Vascular resistance
- ↓ Lipid catabolism
- ↓ Vascular elasticity = ↑ DBP
- ↓ Response to postural stress

Pulmonary

- ↓ Recoil within the lung
- Calcification of soft tissue in the chest wall
- ↓ PO_2 from 20–70 years
- ↓ VO_2 max
- ↓ Pulmonary blood flow = ↓ O_2 Sat
- ↑ RV

Integumentary

- ↓ Thickness with ↑ risk of breakdown
- Uneven pigmentation
- ↓ Vascularity = altered thermoregulation
- ↓ Sub-q tissue ↑ risk for
- Hypothermia

GI

- ↓ Peristalsis
- ↓ Enzymatic activity
- ↓ Motility

Urogenital/Renal

- ↓ Bladder capacity
- ↓ Bladder elasticity
- Prostate hyperplasia
- ↓ Kidney mass
- ↓ Glomerular filtration rate
- ↓ Creatinine clearance

Special Senses

- ↓ Visual acuity
- ↓ Hearing
- ↓ Smell & taste
- ↓ Thymus function
- ↓ Ca^{++} control
- ↓ Sweating

Immune

- ↓ Function/resistance
- ↓ T-cells
- ↓ Temperature regulation

Psychosocial

- ↑ Incidence of depression
- ↑ Fatigue
- Cognitive deficits

Influence of Aging on Laboratory Values

	Test	Aging Influence
Chemistry	AST, ALT	No change
	Alkaline phosphatase	↑ 20% males; ↑ 37% females
	GGTP, serum bilirubin	No change
	Serum albumin	Slight ↓
	Serum magnesium	↑ 15% from 30-80 yrs
	Uric acid	Slight ↓
Lipids	Total cholesterol	30-40mg/dL ↑ by 55 yrs in females & 60 yrs in males
	HDL cholesterol	30% ↓ in males; 30% ↓ in females from 30-80 yrs
	Triglycerides	30% ↑ in males; 50% ↑ in females from 30-80 yrs
Gases	pH	No change
	PaCO₂	No change
	PaO₂	25% ↑ from 30-80 yrs
Renal	Creatinine clearance	10 mL/min/1.73m³/decade
	Serum creatinine	No change
Thyroid	T₃	Slight ↑
	T₄	No change
	Thyrotropin	Slight ↑
Blood	Fasting blood glucose	2 mg/dL per decade > 30 yrs
	ESR (sed rate)	↑ to 40 mm/hr in males & 45 mm/hr in females
	Hematocrit/hemoglobin	No change
	Leukocyte count	Slight ↑
	RBC/platelet count	No change

Source: Brigden ML & Heathcote JC (2000).

Assessment of Falling Risk(s)

Risk Factors for Falling	Yes	No
Have you suffered previous falls?		
Do you have problems with your balance or walking?		
Do you take > 4 of the following medications?		
■ Antipsychotics–Thorazine, Haldol ■ Tricyclic antidepressants–Elavil, Prozac ■ Antianxiety–Valium, Xanax ■ Hypnotics–Seconal, Butulan, Doral ■ Antihypertensives		
Do you have problems with your vision?		
Do you get dizzy when you change positions?		
Do you ever experience light-headedness?		
Are you afraid of falling?		
Do you have problems with your feet?		
Are there hazards around your home that could increase your risk of falling?		
Are your legs weak?		
Is your motion limited in your legs?		
Do you have problems with sensation in your legs?		
Do you have problems thinking clearly?		
Do you have any problems with the following: ■ High blood pressure ■ Arthritis ■ Diabetes ■ Heart disease		

Gait Abnormality Rating Scale–Modified (GARS-M)

Instructions: walk 10 meters at normal pace

Staggering (Partial loss of balance laterally)

0	No loss of balance to the side
1	A single lurch to the side
2	Two lurches to the side
3	Three or more lurches to the side

Arm-Heel Strike Synchrony (Extent of limbs out of phase)

0	Good contralateral arm & leg mov't
1	Arm & leg control out of phase 25% of time
2	Arm & leg control out of phase 25–50% of time
3	Little to no synchrony present

Variability (Consistency & rhythm of steps & arm mov'ts)

0	Fluid & predictably paced limb mov't
1	Occasional changes in velocity (< 25% of time)
2	Unpredictability of rhythm (25–75% of time)
3	Random timing of limb mov'ts

Foot Contact (Heel before forefoot)

0	Very obvious angle of impact of heel
1	Barely visible impact of heel
2	Entire foot striking the ground
3	Anterior foot striking ground before the heel

(Continued text on following page.)

Gait Abnormality Rating Scale–Modified (GARS-M) *(Continued)*

Hip ROM

Obvious hip extension (10°) at double stance	0
Just barely visible hip extension	1
No hip extension	2
Thigh flexion during double stance	3

Shoulder Extension

15° shoulder flexion & 20° shoulder extension	0
Shoulder flexion slightly anterior only	1
Shoulder coming to 0° only with flexion	2
Shoulder staying in extension through the arm swing	3

Guardedness (Hesitancy, slowness, ↓ propulsion)

Good forward momentum & no apprehension	0
COG of HAT (head, arms, trunk) slightly forward in pushoff but good arm-leg coordination	1
HAT held anterior over stance foot; moderate loss of reciprocation	2
HAT held posterior over stance feet; great tenativity in stepping	3

Score of 9.0 = history of falling & 3.8 = no history of falling

Source: Van Swearingen J, Paschal K, Bonino P & Yang J (1996).

Home Safety Checklist	Yes	No
Entrances/exits are well lit		
Lights can be turned on before entering room		
Stairways are well lit		
There is a light within reach of the bed		
Telephone is accessible		
Emergency numbers are posted		
Steps have handrails		
Steps are free of clutter		
Small rugs are tacked down		
Flooring is in good condition		
Door sills are level with floor		
Pathways are free of extension cords		
Pets are out of the pathways		
Bathtub/shower has nonskid surfaces		
Bathtub/shower has grab bar(s)		
A shower chair is available		
Raised toilet seat is available		
Everyday items are stored on lower shelves		
Smoke detectors are in good working order		
Carbon monoxide detectors are present		
Hot water temperature is $\leq 120°$		

Berg Balance Scale

Sitting: Please stand up. Try not to use your hand for support.

(4) Able to stand without using hands & stabilize independently

(3) Able to stand independently using hands

(2) Able to stand using hands after several tries

(1) Needs minimal aid to stand or to stabilize

(0) Needs mod/max assist to stand

Standing to sitting: Please sit down.

(4) Sits safely with minimal use of hands

(3) Controls descent by using hands

(2) Uses back of legs against chair to control descent

(1) Sits independently but has uncontrolled descent

(0) Needs assistance to sit

Stand unsupported: Please stand for 2 min without holding.

(4) Able to stand safely 2 min

(3) Able to stand 2 min w/supervision

(2) Able to stand 30 sec unsupported

(1) Needs several tries to stand 30 sec unsupported

(0) Unable to stand 30 sec unassisted

Transfers: Please transfer from bed/chair to chair (one should have an armrest).

(4) Transfers safely with minor use of hands

(3) Transfers safely with definite need for hands

(2) Transfers w/VC &/or supervision

(1) Needs 1 person to assist

(0) Needs 2 people to assist

Sitting with back unsupported but feet supported on floor: Please sit with arms folded for 2 min.

(4) Able to sit safely 2 min

(3) Able to sit 2 min w/supervision

(2) Able to sit 30 sec

(1) Able to sit 10 sec

(0) Unable to sit 10 sec without support

Standing unsupported with eyes closed: Please close your eyes & stand still for 10 seconds.

(4) Stands 10 sec safely

(3) Stands 10 sec safely w/supervision

(2) Stands 3 sec safely

(1) Unable to keep eyes closed 3 sec but stays steady

(0) Needs help to keep from falling

Berg Balance Scale (Continued)

Standing unsupported with feet together	Reaching forward with outstretched arm while standing	Pick up object from floor from a standing position
Standing unsupported with feet together: Place your feet together & stand without holding.	**Reaching forward with outstretched arm while standing:** Stand with arms at 90° & reach as far forward as possible (record distance of fingertips).	**Pick up object from floor from a standing position:** Pick up shoe or slipper placed in front of your feet.
(4) Independent x 1 min safely	(4) > 25 cm safely	(4) Able to pick up safely & easily
(3) Independent x 1 min w/supervision	(3) > 12 cm safely	(3) Able to pick up w/supervision
(2) Independent but unable to hold for 30 sec	(2) > 5 cm safely	(2) Unable to pick up but reaches 2–5 cm from floor & keeps balance independently
(1) Need help to attain position but can maintain x 15 sec	(1) reaches but needs supervision	(1) Unable to pick up & needs supervision while trying
(0) Need help to attain position & cannot maintain x 15 sec	(0) loses balance while trying	(0) Unable to try/needs assistance to keep from losing balance

Turning to look behind over shoulder while standing	Turn 360°	Placing alternate foot on step while standing unsupported
Turning to look behind over shoulder while standing: Turn to look directly behind you over left shoulder & then right shoulder.	**Turn 360°:** Turn completely around in a full circle, turn in other direction.	**Placing alternate foot on step while standing unsupported:** Place each foot alternately on a step x 4 times.
(4) Looks behind from both sides & wt shifts well	(4) Turns 360° safely in ≤ 4 sec	(4) Independently & safely completes 8 steps in 20 sec
(3) Looks behind from 1 side only, shows less wt shift	(3) Turns 360° safely to 1 side only in ≤ 4 sec	(3) Independently & safely completes 8 steps in > 20 sec
(2) Turns sideways only but maintains balance	(2) Turns 360° safely but slowly	(2) Completes 4 steps w/o w aid with supervision
(1) Needs supervision when turning	(1) Needs close supervision or VC	(1) Completes > 2 steps with min assist
(0) Needs assist to keep from losing balance or falling	(0) Needs assistance while turning	(0) Needs assist to keep from falling

(Continued text on following page)

Berg Balance Scale (Continued)

Standing unsupported one foot in front: Place one foot directly in front of the other & stand for 30 seconds.
(4) Tandem independently & hold 30 sec
(3) Able to place foot ahead of other independently & hold 30 sec
(2) Takes small step independently & holds 30 sec
(1) Needs help to take step but can hold 15 sec
(0) Loses balance while stepping or standing

Stand on one leg: Stand on one leg as long as you can without holding.
(4) Lifts leg independently & holds > 10 sec
(3) Lifts leg independently & holds 5–10 sec
(2) Lifts leg independently & holds ≥ 3 sec
(1) Tries to lift leg, unable to hold 3 sec but remains standing independently
(0) Unable to try or needs assist to prevent fall

Total Score: (maximum = 56)
Score of 45 is the cutoff score for fallers vs. nonfallers.
Sensitivity = 64%
Specificity = 90%

Normative Values for the Berg Balance Scale

Age	Gender	Mean	Range
60–69	Male	55	53-56
60–69	Female	55	51-56
70–79	Male	54	48-56
70–79	Female	53	45-56
80–89	Male	53	49-56
80–89	Female	50	44-56

Source: Berg K, Wood-Dauphinee S & Williams JI (1992).

Tinetti Assessment Tool: Balance

Task	Description	Points	Score
Sitting balance	Leans or slides in chair	0	
	Steady, safe	1	
Arises	Unable without help	0	
	Able, uses arms for help	1	
	Able without using arms	2	
Attempts to arise	Unable without help	0	
	Able, requires >1 attempt	1	
	Able to rise, 1 attempt	2	
Immediate standing balance (first 5 sec)	Unsteady (swaggers), moves feet, trunk sway)	0	
	Steady but uses walker or other support	1	
	Steady without walker or other support	2	
Standing balance	Unsteady	0	
	Steady but wide stance (heels > 4" apart) & uses cane or other support	1	
	Narrow stance without support	2	
Nudged in sitting (examiner pushes lightly on subject's sternum w/ palm of hand)	Begins to fall	0	
	Staggers, grabs, catches self	1	
	Steady	2	
Eyes closed (seated)	Unsteady	0	
	Steady	1	
Turning 360°	Discontinuous steps	0	
	Continuous steps	1	
	Unsteady (grabs, swaggers)	0	
	Steady	1	
Sitting down	Unsafe (misjudged distance, falls into chair)	0	
	Uses arms or not a smooth motion	1	
	Safe, smooth motion	2	
Balance Score			

Tinetti Assessment Tool: Gait

Task	Description	Points	Score
Initiation of gait	Any hesitancy or multiple attempts to start	0	
	No hesitancy	1	
Step length & height	■ R swing foot does not pass L stance foot	0	
	■ R swing foot passes L stance foot	1	
	■ R foot does not clear floor completely with step	0	
	■ R foot completely clears floor	1	
	■ L swing foot does not pass R stance foot	0	
	■ L swing foot passes R stance foot	1	
	■ L foot does not clear floor completely with step	0	
	■ L foot completely clears floor	1	
Step symmetry	R step length ≠ L step length	0	
	R step length = L step length	1	
Step continuity	Stopping or discontinuity between steps	0	
	Steps appear continuous	1	
Path	Marked deviation (1" deviation over 10' course)	0	
	Mild/moderate deviation or uses walking aid	1	
	Straight without walking aid	2	
Trunk	Marked sway or uses walking aid	0	
	No sway but flexion of knees/back, or spreads arms out while walking	1	
	No sway, no flexion, no use of arms, & no use of walking aid	2	
Walking stance	Heels apart	0	
	Heel almost touching while walking	1	

Gait Score

Balance + Gait Score =

Interpretation: 19–24 = at risk for falls
< 19 = at high risk for falls

Source: Tinetti ME (1986).

Timed Up & Go Test (TUG)

Procedure: Phase 1–TUG alone

- Person is seated
- Place visible object 3 meters (~10') away
- Have person get up, walk around object, & sit back down
- Practice once, then time the test 3×

Procedure: Phase 2–TUG cognitive

- Complete phase 1 while counting backward from a randomly selected number between 20 & 100

Procedure: Phase 3–TUG manual

- Complete phase 1 while carrying a full cup of water

Scoring: Individual is at risk for falls if

- TUG alone is ≥ 13.5 seconds (90% correct prediction rate)
- TUG cognitive is ≥ 15 seconds (87% correct prediction rate)
- TUG manual is ≥ 14.5 seconds (90% correct prediction rate)

Mean TUG Scores		
Age & Gender	Without Cane	With Cane
65–69		
Male	9.93 ± 1.40	11.57 ± 1.31
Female	10.15 ± 2.91	14.19 ± 4.67
70–74		
Male	10.45 ± 1.85	12.23 ± 1.88
Female	10.37 ± 2.23	14.27 ± 5.22
75–79		
Male	10.48 ± 1.59	11.82 ± 5.22
Female	10.98 ± 2.68	15.29 ± 5.08

Warning Signs of Elder Abuse

- Bruises, black eyes, welts, lacerations
- Multiple reports of falls/fx
- Open wounds, cuts, punctures, pressure ulcers (untreated in various stages of healing)
- Internal injuries or bleeding
- Broken eyeglasses
- Signs of being restrained (rope marks)
- Multiple trips to the ER
- Depression
- Over- and underutilization of prescribed medications
- Soiled or torn clothing
- Malnutrition/weight loss
- Frequent changes in medical providers
- Sudden change in an elder's behavior
- Confusion attributed to dementia
- A caregiver's refusal to allow visitors to see an elder alone

Musculoskeletal Pathology

Risk Factors for Osteoporosis

- Family hx–if someone in your family has osteoporosis, you have a 60–80% chance of developing the condition. If your mother fx a hip, you have $2\times$ the risk of a hip fx
- Low Ca^{++} intake
  - Child 1–12 yrs = 800 mg/day
  - Teens 13–18 yrs = 700–1200 mg/day
  - Adult = 700–1000 mg/day
  - Pregnant = 1200 mg/day
  - Postmenopausal = 1500 mg/day
- Alcohol, tobacco, & caffeine abuse
- Below normal body weight
- Chronic medical conditions–RA, hyperthyroidism, hyperparathyroidism, DM, liver disease
- Loss of height > 1"
- Sedentary life style
- Early menopause

Substances That Can ↑ Bone Density

- Aluminum
- Antiseizure meds
- Corticosteroids
- Cytotoxic meds
- ↓ Thyroxine
- Heparin
- Caffeine
- Tobacco

Signs & Symptoms of Osteoporosis

- Severe & localized
- ↓ Pain with prolonged T-L–spine pain
- ↑ Pain in hook-lying posture
- ↓ Pain with Valsalva maneuver
- Loss of ht > 1"
- Kyphosis
- Dowager's hump

Signs & Symptoms of Multiple Myeloma

- Recurrent bacterial infections (pneumonia)
- Anemia, weakness, fatigue
- Osteoporosis, spontaneous fx, bone pain
- Kidney stones
- CTS, LBP with radiculopathy

Source: Goodman C & Snyder T (2000).

Arthritic Changes

OA	RA	Gout
■ Asymmetrical involvement	■ Symmetrical jt swelling	■ Affects only a few joints
■ Large wt-bearing joints	■ Small jts–hands, feet, wrist	■ Most common = 1st MTP, knee, wrist
■ Loss of jt surface integrity	■ Erythema & fever	■ Abrupt onset of severe pain
■ Formation of osteophytes	■ Intense pain after rest	■ Uric acid crystals in the synovial fluid
■ Intra-articular loose bodies	■ Wt loss, nutritional deficiencies	■ ↑ Frequency with ↑ age
■ Soft tissue contractures	■ Loss of stamina & weakness	■ Males > females
■ ↓ ROM	■ ↑ Proteolytic enzymes	■ Usually begins @ night
■ Stiffness after activity	■ Enlarged spleen	
■ Deep ache	■ Lymphadenopathy	
	■ Heart & lung pathology	
	■ Jt subluxations	
	■ Vasculitis	
	■ Rheumatoid nodules	

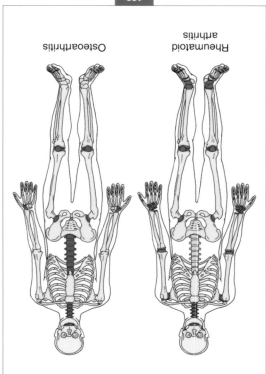

Rheumatoid
arthritis

Osteoarthritis

Neuromuscular Pathology

Modified Ashworth Tone Assessment Scale

0	No ↑ in muscle tone
1	Slight ↑ in muscle tone; catch & release or minimal resistance at end ROM
1+	Slight ↑ in muscle tone; catch, followed by minimal resistance throughout ROM ($< 1/2$)
2	More marked ↑ in muscle tone throughout most of the ROM but affected part is easily moved
3	Considerable ↑ in muscle tone; passive mov't is difficult
4	Affected part is rigid in flexion or extension

Source: Bohannon RW & Smith MB (1986); Ashworth B (1964).

SCI Autonomic Dysreflexia

Exaggerated sympathetic reflex response in SCI patients

- Severe hypertension
- Bradycardia
- Headache
- Vasospasm, skin pallor & gooseflesh below the level of injury
- Arterial vasodilation, flushed skin, & profuse sweating above the level of injury

Neurological Lesions

- Cerebellar = ↓ postural control, ataxia, intention tremor, nystagmus, dysmetria, dysdiadochokinesia, dysphagia, dysarthria
- Basal ganglia = bradykinesia, resting tremor
- Subthalamic nucleus = ballismus
- Caudate & putamen = athetoid
- Globus pallidus = ↓ spontaneous mov't (parkinsonism)

Normal Pressure Hydrocephalus

Sometimes misdiagnosed in a population > 60 yo as part of aging, Alzheimer's or parkinsonism. Symptoms include:

- Gait disturbance–wide BOS, slow/shuffling steps
- Dementia, forgetfulness, short-term memory loss
- Urinary frequency (every 1–2 hrs) → incontinence

Vestibular Disorders

- Chief symptom is rotational vertigo with mov't of the head
- Postural imbalance
- Nausea
- Nystagmus

Guillain-Barré Syndrome (GBS)

Progressive demyelination of peripheral nerves resulting from an autoimmune response. Often occurs after viral or URI
Onset: Effects all ages but peaks 15–35 & 50–75 yo
♂ > ♀ 1.5:1

Signs & Symptoms

- Weakness–symmetrical LE > UE > respiratory
- Paresthesia starts in toes & progress proximal (no loss of sensation)
- Asymmetrical facial weakness, dysphasia, dysarthrias
- Unstable vital signs
- ↓ Reflexes
- Hypotonia
- Fever, nausea, fatigue
- Pain = LB & buttocks
- Cranial nerves affected in 45–75% of cases

Myasthenia Gravis

Myasthenia gravis comes from the Greek & Latin words meaning "grave muscular weakness." It is an immune problem with acetylcholine receptors blocked.
Primary onset: 20–30 yo ♀ > ♂ & > 50 ♂ > ♀

Signs & Symptoms

- Diplopia & ptosis = most common symptoms
- Proximal muscle weakness
- Cranial nerve weakness
- Problem controlling eye mov't & facial expressions
- Difficulty swallowing & chewing
- Dysarthria/dysphagia
- Change in voice quality
- No sensory changes
- No change in DTRs

The edrophonium chloride (Tensilon) test is performed by injecting this chemical into a vein. Improvement of strength immediately after the injection provides strong support for the diagnosis of MG.

Parkinson's Disease

Primary onset = 5th – 6th decade
Affects > 1 in 100 people over the age of 75 yrs
Expect 1.5 million people living with PD in USA by 2020

Primary Signs & Symptoms	Secondary Signs & Symptoms
- Vague unilateral weakness - Muscular rigidity - Resting tremor (pill rolling) - Bradykinesia → akinesia - Cogwheel rigidity - Impaired postural reflexes (loss of balance): disturbance of spatial organization, dependence on visual input for balance - Tight facial appearance (parkinsonian mask) - Cognitive decline - Depression/panic attacks - Gait abnormalities: ↓ step length & arm swing, festination of gait (inability to stop) - Micrographia (handwriting becomes small)	- Dementia - Vital capacity declines - Poorly localized pain - Paresthesia - ↓ Autonomic control - Sweating - Drooling (sialorrhea) due to abnormal swallow - Loss of volume & emotion in voice - Reduced libido - Inability to stay asleep

Source: Parkinson's Disease Handbook (2004).

Hoehn & Yahr Staging of Parkinson's Disease

Stage 1
- Signs & symptoms are mild & unilateral
- Symptoms are inconvenient but not disabling
- Usually presents with tremor of one limb
- Friends notice changes in posture, locomotion, & facial expression

Stage 2
- Symptoms are bilateral
- Minimal disability
- Posture & gait affected but no impairment of balance

Stage 3
- Significant slowing of body movements
- Early impairment of equilibrium with walking or standing
- Generalized dysfunction that is moderately severe but patient can still be independent

Stage 4
- Severe symptoms
- Can still walk to a limited extent
- Rigidity & bradykinesia
- No longer able to live alone (requires help for ADLs)
- Tremor may be less than earlier stages

Stage 5
- Cachectic stage
- Invalidism complete
- Cannot stand or walk
- Requires constant nursing care

Source: Hoehn MM & Yahr MD (1967).

Stages of Alzheimer's Disease

Stage 1: No cognitive impairment

- No memory problems

Stage 2: Very mild decline

- Individual reports memory lapses–forgetting words, names, location of everyday objects
- Problems are not evident to medical professional, friends, family

Stage 3: Mild decline

- Problem with memory or concentration may be measurable in clinical testing
- Friends, family, coworkers notice deficiencies
- Common difficulties include word-finding problems, decreased ability to remember names when introduced to new people, poor reading retention, losing/misplacing valuable objects, decreased ability to plan or organize

Stage 4: Moderate decline (mild or early-stage Alzheimer's disease)

- Deficiencies noted in medical interview
- Decreased knowledge of recent occasions or current events
- Impaired ability to perform challenging mental math–count backwards from 100 by 7s
- Decreased capacity to perform complex tasks–planning dinner for guests, paying bills, etc
- Reduced memory of personal history
- Individual may be subdued & withdrawn in socially or mentally challenging situations

Stage 5: Moderately severe decline (moderate or mid-stage Alzheimer's disease)

- Major gaps in memory & deficits in cognitive function
- Assistance needed in day-to-day activities
- Unable to recall address, telephone number, name of school graduated
- Confused about time, day of week, season
- Has trouble with less challenging mental math–count backward from 40 by 4s or from 20 by 2s
- Usually retains knowledge about self, names of spouse & children
- Usually does not require assistance with eating or toileting

Stage 6: Severe decline (moderately severe or mid-stage Alzheimer's disease)

- Significant personality changes, hallucinations or compulsive behaviors may emerge
- Loss of awareness of recent experiences
- Generally recalls own name & distinguishes familiar faces but may forget the name of spouse, caregiver
- Needs helps with ADLs & toileting; disruption in sleep/wake cycle
- Tends to wander and become lost

Stage 7: Very severe decline (severe or late-stage Alzheimer's disease)

- Loss of ability to respond to the environment & the ability to control mov't
- Speech becomes unrecognizable
- Needs help with eating (difficulty swallowing); generally incontinent
- Loss of ability to ambulate without assistance
- Poor muscle control, abnormal reflexes, muscle rigidity

Source: Alzheimer's Association.

Mini Mental State Examination (MMSE)

Score	Maximum	Task
	5	**Orientation:** What is the (year) (season) (date) (day) (month)?
	5	Where are we (state) (country) (town) (building) (floor)?
	3	**Registration:** Name 3 objects: 1 second to say each. Ask the patient all 3 after you have said them. Give 1 pt for each correct answer. Repeat them until he/she learns all 3. Count & record trials: _____
	5	**Attention & Calculation:** Serial 7s. Score 1 point for each correct answer. Stop after 5 answers (Alternative question: Spell "world" backward)
	3	**Recall:** Ask for the 3 objects repeated above. Give 1 point for each correct answer.
	2	**Language:** Name a pencil & watch
	1	Repeat the following "No, ifs, ands, or buts"
	3	Follow a 3-stage command: "Take a paper in your hand, fold it in half, & put it on the floor."
	1	Read & obey the following: "Close your eyes."
	1	Write a sentence
	1	Copy the design shown: 
	30	**Total score (Normal ≥ 24)**

Source: Folstein MF, Folstein SE & McHugh PR (1975).

Cardiovascular & Pulmonary Pathology

Wells Clinical Score for Deep Vein Thrombosis

Clinical Parameter Score	Score
Active cancer (treatment ongoing or within 6 months)	+ 1
Paralysis or recent plaster immobilization of LE	+ 1
Recently bedridden for >3 days or major surgery < 4 weeks	+ 1
Localized tenderness along the distribution of the deep venous system	+ 1
Entire leg swelling	+ 1
Calf swelling > 3 cm compared to asymptomatic leg	+ 1
Pitting edema (> asymptomatic leg)	+ 1
Previous DVT documented	+ 1
Collateral superficial veins (nonvaricose)	+ 1
Alternative diagnosis (as likely or > that of DVT)	− 2

Total Score	
High probability	≥ 3
Moderate probability	1 – 2
Low probability	≤ 0

Source: Anand SS, Wells PS, Hunt D, et al. (1998).

Additional Risks of DVT

- AIDS
- Long airline flights
- Varicose veins
- Recent central venous catheterization
- Pacemakers
- Blood type A
- Pregnancy
- Antithrombin deficiency
- Obesity
- Oral contraceptives
- Acute MI

Transient Ischemic Attack (TIA)

Symptoms depend on cerebral vessel involved

- Anterior Cerebral Artery = LE > UE; frontal signs
- Middle Cerebral Artery = forearm, hand, & mouth affected
- Posterior Cerebral Artery = visual disturbances, graying out, blurring, fogging

Signs & Symptoms of a Pulmonary Embolus

- Anginalike pain or crushing chest pain
- Dyspnea, wheezing, rales
- ↓ BP
- Hemoptysis, chronic cough
- Fever
- Tachypnea (> 16/min)
- Tachycardia (> 100/min)
- Diaphoresis

Clinical Signs of Hypertension

- Spontaneous epistaxis
- Occipital h/a
- Dizziness
- Visual changes
- Nocturnal urinary frequency
- Flushed face

Source: Goodman C & Snyder T (2000).

Peripheral Arterial Occlusive Disease

- > 60 yo
- Hx of DM, heart disease, smoking
- Cool LEs
- ↓ Capillary refill
- Ankle-Brachial Index < 0.80

Signs & Symptoms of Leukemia

- Epistaxis, bleeding gums
- Hematuria, rectal bleeding
- Bruising of the skin, petechiae
- Infections, fever
- Weakness, fatigue
- Enlarged lymph nodes
- Weight loss, loss of appetite
- Enlarged spleen

Source: Goodman C & Snyder T (2000).

Effects of Dehydration

Causes

- ↓ CNS function with ↓ thirst
- Vomiting/diarrhea
- DM
- Excess sweating / fever
- Surgery
- Medications (diuretics)

Signs & Symptoms

- Altered mentation
- Lethargy/agitation
- Light-headedness/syncope
- Orthostatic hypotension
- Weakness

Pneumonia

- One of the most common causes of death in the elderly
- Typical symptoms
  - Productive cough (rust-colored sputum)
  - Fever, chills
  - Pleuritic chest pain
  - SOB
- Additional symptoms
  - Confusion
  - CHF
  - Anorexia
  - Change in sleep habits

Tuberculosis

Populations at Risk

- Homeless
- Health-care workers
- Inmates
- Immunocompromised
- > 65 years of age
- Injection drug user
- Malnourished

Signs & Symptoms

- Fatigue
- Anorexia
- Low-grade fever
- Night sweats
- Frequent/productive cough
- Dyspnea
- Avascular necrosis of hip

Integumentary Pathology

Braden Scale for the Risk of Pressure Ulcers

Risk Factor	1	2	3	4	Score
Sensory Perception—Ability to respond meaningfully to pressure-related discomfort	Completely limited	Very limited	Slightly limited	No impairment	
Moisture—Extent to which skin is exposed to moisture	Completely moist	Moist	Occasionally moist	Rarely moist	
Activity—Amount of physical activity	Bedfast	Chair fast	Walks occasionally	Walks frequently	
Mobility—Ability to change or control body position	Completely immobile	Very limited	Slightly limited	No limitations	
Nutrition—Usual food intake pattern	Very poor	Probably inadequate	Adequate	Excellent	
Friction & Shear	Problem	Potential problem	No apparent problem		
The lower the score, the higher the risk of a pressure ulcer					

Source: http://www.bradenscale.com/braden.PDF

Clinical Presentation of Venous vs. Arterial Ulcers

Venous Ulceration	Feature	Arterial Ulceration
Family hx, previous DVT	Risks	Smoking, DM, ↑ cholesterol, HTN
40–60 yrs old	Age	> 60 yrs old
Women	Gender	Men
Medial LE	Site	Malleoli, heel, 5th metatarsal base, toes
Present; ↑ with elevation	Pain	Severe; ↑ with dependency
Irregular	Margins	Regular; appears "punched out"
Pink & granulated	Base	Necrotic & no granulation
Present, often significant	Swelling	Absent
Warm	Temperature	Cool to cold
Present	Pulses	Decreased or absent
Venous staining	Adjacent skin	Shiny, thick nails, hair loss

Ankle—Brachial Index: Right Ankle SBP/Right Brachial SBP

> 0.96	Normal
> 0.95	Abnormal (mild disease)
> 0.80	Probable claudication (moderate disease)
> 0.50	Moderate-severe disease
> 0.30	Ischemia, tissue necrosis, severe disease

Staging of Pressure Ulcers

Stage 1: A defined area of persistent redness in lightly pigmented skin & persistent red, blue, or purple hues in darker skin. Changes in skin temperature, tissue consistency, &/or sensation may be present as compared to adjacent areas.

Stage 2: Partial-thickness skin loss of the epidermis &/or dermis. The ulcer is superficial & presents as an abrasion, blister, or shallow crater.

Stage 3: Full-thickness skin loss with damage/necrosis of sub-q tissue into fascia. Presents as a deep crater with or without undermining.

Stage 4: Full-thickness skin loss with extensive destruction/ necrosis to muscle, bone, tendon, or jt capsule. Undermining & sinus tracts may also be present.

Eschar: Thick, dry, black necrotic tissue–not staged.

Source: AHCPR Publication # 92-0050.

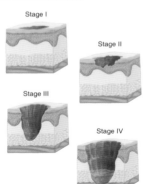

Stage I

Stage II

Stage III

Stage IV

	Pressure Ulcer A-S-S-E-S-S-M-E-N-T Tool	
A	Anatomic location	Sacrum, heel, trochanter, lateral malleolus, ischium, elbow (R/L)
S	Size	Measure: length, width, depth Shape Stage I, II, III, IV, not staged
S	Sinus tract, tunneling, undermining	Present—Not present Location: _____ o'clock
E	Exudate	Color: serous–sanguineous Amount: scant, moderate, copious Consistency: clear–purulent
S	Sepsis	Infection: local, systemic, none
S	Surrounding skin	Dark, discolored, erythematous, intact, swollen
M	Margins	Edges: attached, not attached, rolled
E	Erythema	Present–not present Epithelialization: present–not present Eschar: yellow slough, black, soft, hard, stringy Surrounding area: dry, moist, red
N	Necrotic tissue	Present—not present Nose (Odor): present–not present New blood vessels: present–not present
T	Tissue bed	Granulation tissue: present–not present Tenderness: pain–no pain Medication: yes–no Tension: tautness/hard–not hard Temperature: warm, cool, normal

Source: Ayello EA (1996).

Cellulitis

A serious bacterial infection of the skin that can spread to lymph nodes & bloodstream. Cellulitis is not contagious.

People at Risk

- DM
- Circulatory px
- Liver disease
- Eczema
- Psoriasis
- Chickenpox
- Severe acne
- Hx of CHF

Signs & Symptoms

- Pain, swelling, warmth
- Erythema with streaks & vague borders
- Fever & chills
- Recent skin disruption
- Headache
- Low BP
- Enlarged lymph nodes
- Small red spots appear on top of reddened skin

Herpes Zoster (Shingles)

- 2/3 of patients are > 50 yo
- Pain, tenderness, & paraesthesia in the dermatome may be present 3–5 days before vesicular eruption
- Prodromal pain may mimic cardiac or pleural pain
- Erythema & vesicles follow a dermatomal distribution
- Pustular vesicles from crusts lasting 2–3 weeks
- Thoracic (50%) & ophthalmic division of trigeminal nerve are most commonly affected regions
- Contagious via respiratory droplets or direct contact with blisters

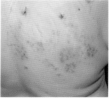

Source: From Barankin B & Freiman A (2006).

Gastrointestinal Pathology

Bowel Pathology

Colon/Rectal Cancer	Irritable Bowel	Inflammatory Bowel (Crohn's or Ulcerative Colitis)
■ Hemorrhoids	■ Affects females in early adulthood	■ Joint arthralgia
■ Rectal bleeding	■ Stress related	■ Skin lesions (ankles, shins)
■ Back pain referred to LES	■ Variable/intermittent S&S	■ Light sensitivity
■ Change in bowel patterns	■ Abdominal cramps	■ ↓ Pain with gas/BM
■ Nausea & vomiting	■ Nausea & vomiting	■ Anemia due to blood loss
■ Fatigue & dyspnea due to iron deficiency	■ Flatulence	■ Wt loss
■ Wt loss	■ Change in bowel patterns	■ Clubbing of fingers
■ Red/mahogany stools	■ Foul breath	■ Fever
		■ Rectal bleeding
		■ (+) Psoas test

Hepatic Pathology

Hepatitis

Generalized Signs & Symptoms:

- Nausea
- Vomiting
- Low-grade fever/chills
- Loss of appetite
- Lethargy

- Jaundice—skin & eyes
- Liver pain
- Dark urine
- Light-colored stools

Type	Incubation	Transmission	Cause
A	15–45 days	Fecal-oral (does not develop into chronic hepatitis)	Contaminated milk, water, shellfish, unsanitary conditions
B	2–3 months	Blood or body fluids Infants = carriers (can become chronic)	Contaminated needles, transfusion
C	15–90 days	Blood or body fluids (can become chronic)	Transfusion
D	25–75 days	Blood or body fluids	Occurs in presence of Hep B, IV drug use
E	20–80 days	Fecal-oral	Contaminated milk, water, shellfish
G	Unknown	Blood or body fluids	Transfusion, IV drug use

Endocrine Pathology

Hyperthyroidism (Graves' Disease)

Signs & Symptoms in Order of Frequency:

Patients ≥ 70 years of age	Patients ≤ 50 years of age
■ Tachycardia	■ Tachycardia
■ Fatigue	■ Hyperactive reflexes
■ Weight loss	■ ↑ Sweating
■ Tremor	■ Heat intolerance
■ Dyspnea	■ Fatigue
■ Apathy	■ Tremor
■ Anorexia	■ Nervousness
■ Nervousness	■ Polydipsia
■ Hyperactive reflexes	■ Weakness
■ Weakness	■ ↑ Appetite
■ Depression	■ Dyspnea
■ ↑ Sweating	■ Weight loss
■ Polydipsia	■ Diarrhea
■ Diarrhea	■ Apathy
■ Confusion	■ Depression
■ Muscular atrophy	■ Muscular atrophy
■ Heat intolerance	■ Anorexia
■ Constipation	

Source: Trivalle C, et al. (1996).

Hypothyroidism

- ■ ↓ Basal metabolic rate
- ■ Dry skin
- ■ Muscle/joint pain
- ■ Proximal weakness
- ■ Lethargy, depression, apathy
- ■ Confusion
- ■ Weight gain
- ■ Edema around the eyes
- ■ Loss of lateral eyebrow
- ■ Cardiomegaly
- ■ Constipation
- ■ Cold intolerance
- ■ Brittle nails
- ■ Sparse/coarse hair
- ■ Peripheral edema
- ■ Jt effusion with Ca^{++} deposits
- ■ CTS
- ■ Slow healing
- ■ Hoarseness
- ■ PR < 60 in untrained person

Gout

- Rapid onset of sudden severe pain
- Inflammation of 1st MTP, knee, wrist, or elbow
- Redness, swelling
- Tenderness, hypersensitivity
- Fever, chills
- Yellowish-white papules on the fingertips, ears, elbows, & knuckles
- Note: Some diuretics used to treat CHF can cause gout.

Diabetes Mellitus

↑ Signs & Symptoms

- ↑ Urination
- ↑ Thirst
- ↑ Hunger
- ↑ Fatigue/lethargy
- Numbness/tingling feet/hands

Complications

- Blindness
- Glaucoma
- Cataracts
- H/A
- Stroke
- Foot ulcers
- Kidney disease

Abnormal Blood Glucose

Hypoglycemia	Hyperglycemia
■ Blood glucose < 50–60 mg/dL	■ Blood glucose > 180 mg/dL
■ Skin is pale, cool, diaphoretic	■ Skin is dry & flushed
■ Disoriented or agitated	■ Fruity breath odor
■ Headache	■ Blurred vision
■ Blurred vision	■ Dizziness
■ Slurred speech	■ Weakness
■ Tachycardic with palpitations	■ Nausea
■ Weak/shaky	■ Vomiting
■ Lip/tongue numbness	■ Cramping
■ LOC	■ Increased urination
	■ LOC/seizure

Urogenital Pathology

5 Major Signs & Symptoms of Urinary Tract Pathology

1. Blood in urine (hematuria)
2. Edema–fluid retention
3. Pain–percussion over kidneys
4. Enlargement of kidneys
5. Anemia

Factors that Contribute to Urinary Incontinence

- UTIs
- Vaginal infection
- Constipation
- Medications
- Childbirth
- Surgery or trauma

- Normal pressure hydrocephalus
- Weak bladder muscles
- Overactive bladder muscles
- Enlarged prostate
- Damage to nerves of the bladder, i.e., MS, Parkinson's

Types of Urinary Incontinence

- Stress incontinence: occurs when urine leaks during exercise, coughing, sneezing, laughing, lifting; most common in young or middle-aged women when pelvic muscle are weakened by childbirth or surgery
- Urge incontinence: urge comes on quickly & unable to get to the toilet in time; common in people who have had a CVA, DM, or Alzheimer's, Parkinson's, MS
- Overflow incontinence: constant urine dripping due to an overfull bladder; common in SCI, DM, & prostate px
- Functional incontinence: occurs in the disabled or aging patient when mobility limits the ability to get to the toilet in time

Benign Prostate Hyperplasia (BPH)

Signs & Symptoms

- Impaired emptying or residual urine retention
- Reduced caliber of force of urine stream
- Difficulty starting urine stream

Prostate cancer–PSA > 4 ng/mL (see Other Pathology—
Metastatic tumors)

Other Pathology

Lymphoma

- Swollen lymph nodes in neck & axilla
- Malaise & weight loss
- Fever & night sweats
- Itching

Non-Hodgkin's Lymphoma

- Peak incidence is 20–24 yrs of age
- Appearance of swollen glands in neck, axilla, groin
- Nonpainful & unresponsive to antibiotics
- Loss of appetite, nausea, vomiting, indigestion, wt loss
- Enlargement of liver, spleen, abdominal lymph nodes
- LBP referred to LE
- Anemia
- Night sweats & recurring fevers

Signs & Symptoms Associated with the Most Common Primary Sites of Metastatic Tumors

Lung*	Prostate	Renal	Breast	Colon
■ > 60 yrs old ■ Smoker ■ Shoulder, chest & C-spine pain ■ TOS symptoms ■ Chronic cough ■ Bloody sputum ■ Malaise ■ Wt loss ■ Fever ■ Dyspnea ■ Wheezing	■ > 50 yrs old ■ L/S pain ■ Frequent urination ■ Weak urine stream ■ Difficulty starting urination	■ 55–60 yrs old ■ Hematuria ■ Wt loss ■ Malaise ■ Fever ■ Palpable posterior lateral abdominal mass	■ 20–50 yrs old & > 65 yrs old ■ Nipple pain ■ Nipple discharge ■ Dimpling of breast ■ Palpable mass	■ > 50 yrs old ■ Abdominal pain ■ L/S pain ■ Change in bowel habits ■ Bloody stools ■ Malaise ■ Wt loss ■ Pain unaffected by position

Note: Screening for metastasis to the spine can be done by attempting to provoke a sharp, localized pain with percussion with a reflex hammer over the spinous processes.

*Pancoast tumor-mimics Thoracic Outlet Syndrome, pain in ulnar distribution, intrinsic hand atrophy, UE venous distention

Source: Boissannault WG & Bass C (1990).

References

- AHCPR Publication # 92–0050, Pressure Ulcers in Adults: Prediction & Prevention.
- Ahmed SM & Swedlund SK. evaluation & treatment of urinary tract infections in children. *American Family Physician*. 57(7):1583, 1998.
- American Cancer Society: The Dangers of Tobacco. *Patient Medical Assistant*, August 23, 1999.
- American Lyme Disease Foundation.
- American Physical Therapy Association. Guide to Physical Therapist Practice. Second Edition. *Physical Therapy* 81(1): 9–746, 2001.
- Anand SS, Wells PS, Hunt D, et al. Does this patient have deep vein thrombosis? *JAMA*, 279(14):1094–1099, 1998.
- Asbill CS. Play with steroids, pay the price. *Sports Medicine & Performance*, 3:14–15, 2005.
- Ashworth B. Preliminary trial of carisoprodol in multiple sclerosis. *Practitioner*, 192:540, 1964.
- Atwater SW, Crowe TK, Deitz JC & Richardson PK. Interrater & test-retest reliability of two pediatric balance tests. *Physical Therapy*, 70(2):79–87, 1990.
- Ayello Elizabeth A. A pressure ulcer A-S-S-E-S-S-M-E-N-T Tool, *Nursing*, 26(10):62–63, 1996.
- Bates B. A Guide to Physical Examination, 6th ed. Lippincott, Philadelphia, 1995.
- Berg K, Wood-Dauphinee S & Williams JI. The Balance Scale: Reliability assessment for elder residents & patients with an acute stroke. *Scandinavian Journal of Rehabilitation Medicine*, 27:27–36, 1995.
- Berg K, Wood-Dauphinee S, Williams JI, Holliday P, Maki B. Measuring balance in the elderly: Validity of an instrument. *Canadian Journal of Public Health*, July/August supplement 2:S7–S11, 1992.
- Bohannon RW & Smith MB. Interrater reliability of a modified Ashworth scale of muscle spasticity. *Physical Therapy*, 67:206–207, 1986.
- Boissonnault WG. Primary Care for the Physical Therapist, Philadelphia: Elsevier Saunders, 2005.
- Boissannault WG & Bass C. Pathological origins of trunk & neck pain: Part I: pelvic & abdominal visceral disorders.

Journal of Orthopaedic & Sports Physical Therapy, 12(5); 192–207, 1990.

■ Boissannault WG & Bass C. Pathological origins of trunk & neck pain: Part II–disorders of the cardiovascular & pulmonary systems. *Journal of Orthopaedic & Sports Physical Therapy,* 12(5):208–215, 1990.

■ Boissannault WG & Bass C. Pathological origins of trunk & neck pain: Part III–diseases of the musculoskeletal system, *Journal of Orthopaedic & Sports Physical Therapy,* 12(5):216–221, 1990.

■ Brigden ML & Heathcote JC. Problems in interpreting laboratory tests. *Postgraduate Medicine,* 107(7):145–146, 151–152, 2000.

■ Buskila D, Neumann L, Vaisber G, et al. Increased rates of fibromyalgia following cervical spine injury. A controlled study of 161 cases of traumatic injury, *Arthritis & Rheumatism,* 40(3):446–452, 1997.

■ Ciccone CD. Pharmacology in Rehabilitation, 3rd ed. FA Davis, Philadelphia, 2002.

■ Cox JL, Holden JM & Sagovsky R. Development of the 10-item Edinburgh postnatal depression scale. *British Journal of Psychiatry,* 150:782–786, 1987.

■ Folstein MF, Folstein SE & McHugh PR. Mini-mental state. *Journal of Psychiatric Research,* 12(3):189–198, 1975.

■ Franjoine MR, Gunther JS & Taylor MJ. Pediatric balance scale: a modified version of the Berg balance scale for the school-age child with mild to moderate motor impairment. *Pediatric Physical Therapy,* 15:114–128, 2003

■ Gagnon I, Swaine B, Friedman D & Forget R. Children show decreased dynamic balance after mild traumatic brain injury. *Archives of Physical Medicine & Rehabilitation,* 85:444–452, 2004.

■ Sports Science Exchange. Caffeine Consumption. Chicago, IL, Gatorade Sports Science Institute, 1990.

■ Gawkrodger DJ. Dermatology. 3rd ed. Churchill Livingstone, Edinburgh, 2003.

■ Goodman CC & Boissonnault WG. Pathology: Implications for the Physical Therapist, Philadelphia: WB Saunders, 1998.

- Goodman C & Snyder T. Differential Diagnosis in Physical Therapy, 3rd ed. WB Saunders, Philadelphia, 2000.
- Gulick DT. OrthoNotes. FA Davis, Philadelphia, 2005.
- Guzman J, Burgos-Vargas R, Duarte-Salazar C & Gomez-Mora. Reliability of the articular examination in children with juvenile rheumatoid arthritis. *Journal of Rheumatism,* 22(12):2331–2236, 1995.
- Hirschfeld RM, Williams JB, Spitzer RL, et al. Development and validation of a screening instrument for bipolar spectrum disorder: the Mood Disorder Questionnaire. *American Journal of Psychiatry,* 157(11);1873–1875, 2000.
- Hoehn MM & Yahr MD. Parkinsonism: Onset, progression, & mortality. *Neurology,* 17:427, 1967.
- Hoyert DL, Kung HC & Smith BL. Deaths: Preliminary data for 2003. *National Vital Statistics Report,* 53(15), Hyattsville, Maryland, National Center for Health Statistics, 2005.
- Is AA for you? Twelve questions only you can answer. New York: A.A. World Services, Inc., 1973.
- Jaffer SN & Qureshi AA. Dermatology Quick Glance. New York: McGraw-Hill, 2004.
- Kroumpouzos G. & Cohen L.M. Specific dermatoses of pregnancy: An evidence-based systematic review. *American Journal of Obstetrics & Gynecology,* 188(4):1083–1092, 2003.
- Melzack R. The McGill Pain Questionnaire. In: Pain Measurement & Assessment. New York: Raven Press, 1983 pp 41–48.
- Melzack R. The short-form McGill pain questionnaire. *Pain,* 30:191–197, 1987.
- Munro J & Campbell I (eds). Macleod's Clinical Examination, 10th ed. Philadelphia: Churchill Livingstone, 2000.
- McSweeney JC, Cody M, O'Sullivan P, Elberson K, Moser DK & Garvin BJ. Women's early warning symptoms of acute myocardial infarction. *Circulation,* 108(21);2619–2623, 2003.
- Myers E. LPN Notes: Nurse's Clinical Pocket Guide. Philadelphia: FA Davis, 2004.
- Myers E & Hopkins T. Med Surg Notes: Nurse's Clinical Pocket Guide. Philadelphia: FA Davis, 2004.
- National Institute of Child Health & Human Development, Autism Facts.

- Nunn I & Gregg AJ. Peak expiratory flow in normals. *British Medical Journal*, 3(5874):282–284, 1973.
- Parkinson's Disease Handbook, American Parkinson Disease Assoc., printed by Novartis Pharmaceuticals, 2004.
- Porth CM. Pathophysiology: Concepts of Altered Health States, 4th ed. Philadelphia: JB Lippincott, 1994.
- Purtilo DT. A Survey of Human Diseases. Reading, Mass.: Addison-Welsey Publishing Co Inc, 1978.
- Ransford AO, Cairns D & Mooney V. The pain drawing as an aid to the physical evaluation of patients with low back pain. *Spine*, 1(1), 1976.
- Reddy, S, Latex allergies. *American Family Physician*. 57(1) 93–106.
- Rothstein JM, Roy SH & Wolf SL. Rehabilitation Specialist's Handbook, 3rd ed. Philadelphia: FA Davis, 2005.
- Rubin E & Farber JL. Pathology, 2nd ed. Philadelphia: JB Lippincott, 1994.
- Siegel B. Diagnostic & Statistical Manual of Mental Disorders, 4th ed. Helping Children with Autism Learn, Oxford University Press, 2003.
- Tinetti ME. Performance-oriented assessment of mobility problems in elderly patients. *Journal of the American Geriatrics Society*, 34:119–126, 1986.
- Trivalle C, Doucet J, Chassagne P, Landrin I, Kadri N, Menard JF & Bercoff E. Differences in the signs & symptoms of hyperthyroidism in older & younger patients, *Journal of the American Geriatrics Society*, 44(1):50–53, 1996.
- Urbano FL. Signs of hypocalcemia: Chvostek's & Trousseau's signs. *Hospital Physician*, March, 43–45, 2000.
- Van Swearingen J, Paschal K, Bonino P & Yang J. The modified gait abnormality rating scale for recognizing the risk of recurrent falls in community-dwelling elderly adults. *Physical Therapy*, 76(9):994–1002, 1996.
- Vegso IJ & JS Torg. Field evaluation & management of intracranial injuries. Athletic injuries to the head, neck & face. St. Louis: Mosby-Year Book: 226–227, 1991.
- Waddell G, McCulloch JA, Kummel E & Venner RM. Nonorganic physical signs in low-back pain. *Spine*, 5(2):117–125, 1980.
- Young W. Spinal Cord Injury Levels & Classification. W.M. Keck Center for Collaborative Neuroscience, Rutgers University, Piscataway, NJ, 2001.

- http://www.parenting.ivillage.com (accessed April 19, 2005)
- http://www.nncc.org (accessed April 19, 2005)
- http://www.nofas.org (accessed April 19, 2005)
- http://www.whonamedit.com (accessed April 19, 2005)
- http://www.elderabusecenter.org (accessed June 6, 2005)
- http://www.bradenscale.com/braden.PDF (accessed June 6, 2005)
- http://www.alz.org (accessed April 20, 2005)
- http://www.niams.nih.gov/hi/topics/lupus/slehandout/ (accessed June 11, 2006)
- http://www.myasthenia.org/information/FactsAboutMG.htm (accessed June 11, 2005)
- http://www.alsa.org (accessed June 11, 2005)
- http://CAonline.AmCancerSoc.org (accessed June 12, 2005)
- http://womenshealth.about.com (accessed April 26, 2005)
- http://hcdz.bupa.co.uk/fact.sheets/html/kidney_stones.html (accessed April 26, 2005)
- http://www.marfan.org/ (accessed July 10, 2005)
- http://www.ocfoundation.org/ (accessed July 10, 2005)
- http://www.adhdhelp.net/ (accessed July 10, 2005)
- http://www.patientcenters.com/leukemia/news/signs.html (accessed July 10, 2005)
- www.aldf.com/Lyme.asp (accessed April 19, 2005)
- www.unmc.edu/olson/student/Powerpoints/Physiological%20 Changes%20in%20Pregnancy.ppt (accessed June 30, 2005)
- http://www.andrews.edu/NUFS/caffeine.html (accessed August 14, 2005)
- http://www.afp.org/afp/991101ap/2027.html (accessed August 14, 2005)
- http://www.woundconsultant.com/preview/sitebuilder/staging. pdf (accessed August 28, 2005)
- http://www.npuap.org/positn6.html (accessed August 28, 2005)
- http://www.infantrefluxdisease.com (accessed September 4, 2005)
- http://folsomobgyn.com/placental_abruption.htm (accessed September 4, 2005)
- http://www.skincancer.org (accessed September 30, 2005)

Index

599214219

...fessionals can refer to for the delivery of safe and effective health care.

Organized by life span, **Screening Notes** is a quick and user-friendly tool for all health-care providers, regardless of practice setting. **Screening Notes** provides a guide to effective screening for medical pathologies and co-morbidities that may profoundly influence therapeutic management or fall outside the scope of practice.

Look for our other Davis's Notes titles

Visit us at www.FADavis.com
F.A. Davis Company
Independent Publishers Since 1879

ISBN 10: 0-8036-1573-6
ISBN 13: 978-0-8036-1573-1